Fitness

For
Health,
Figure/Physique,
Posture

Fitness

For Health, Figure/Physique, Posture

Fifth Edition

Ruth Lindsey
California State University
Long Beach

Billie J. Jones
Florida State University
Tallahassee

Ada Van Whitley
Oklahoma State University
Stillwater

wcb

Wm. C. Brown Co. Publishers
2460 Kerper Blvd.
Dubuque, IA 52001

PHYSICAL EDUCATION

Consulting Editor

Aileene Lockhart
Texas Woman's University

2-07267-01

Contents

List of Tables

Preface

· *Fitness for Health, Figure/Physique, Posture* is a revision of the text which was formerly titled *Body Mechanics*. In this fifth edition, the authors have designed a book for both men and women. It is aimed primarily at young adults of college age, but it is suitable for high school through middle age.

The emphasis of the text is conveyed in the new title, but the concepts include health related fitness; figure/physique control; weight and fatness control; nutrition; posture (standing, sitting, walking, stair climbing); body mechanics in daily activities (lifting, carrying, pushing, pulling); care of the back; care of the feet; relaxation; pregnancy and menstruation; exercises and training programs (including weight training, jogging, and calisthenics).

This text-workbook is designed primarily for an exercise course. The emphasis is on "do-it-yourself" improvement, with tests and measurements for evaluating present status, together with suggestions for setting personal goals and the means for accomplishing them.

An *Instructor's Handbook* which accompanies this text includes a course outline, additional exercises, and new source material. It comprises suggested methods and materials for testing and teaching—such as stunts, games, demonstrations, references, and equipment—to add variety to the presentations.

We would like to express our gratitude to many of our colleagues who have used prior editions of this text for providing comments and suggestions, many of which have been incorporated in this present edition.

The Authors

Introduction and Assessment

Overheard as the student rushed into the classroom: "(Puff-puff) Gee, I'm out of shape!" Then came the reply: "Yes, and you seem to be out of condition, too!" And therein lies the quandary. Concern for "shape" and physical condition has led the public to spend millions of dollars for hormones, vitamins, diets, pills, secrets of charm, modeling school, isometric ropes, magic pillows, steam cabinets, and massage. Misled by false advertising and exaggerated claims such as "Lose Weight Without Dieting," "Exercise Without Effort," and "Move Inches Without Moving," they have been led down the proverbial path, with little to show for the results except a thinner purse.

Without fanfare, this book attempts to dispel some of the myths while providing the facts about physique and figure improvement, weight control and physical fitness, as well as methods for conserving energy and avoiding strain in everyday tasks. It is designed primarily as a "do-it-yourself" physical improvement course. There are no secrets or magic formulae to give you a better figure/physique, help you reduce, enhance your poise, or improve your physical condition. Success in achieving the goals you set depends upon your willingness to exert yourself—physically and mentally.

As for body mechanics, the human body, which has often been referred to as a "machine," is subject to the same mechanical forces and laws that govern other machines. With its more than 600 muscles and 200 bones, not to mention other tissues, it probably has more moving parts and is considerably more complicated than man-made machines; but with proper care and use, it will outlast most of them. This book is concerned with the care and use of that body for efficient and effective movement. Statistics show that 60-75 percent of college youth have poor body mechanics; 80 percent of all adults are estimated to have foot problems; 90 percent of arch trouble is thought to be due to improper use of the foot; 80 percent of backaches are postural in origin. Good body mechanics do not assure good health, but they do affect our ability to function and the quality of the life we lead.

In the ensuing pages, you will find tests and measurements for assessing your present status in physical fitness, weight, figure/physique, and posture. Charts allow you to compare yourself with others and to estimate your "ideal" weight and measurements. From this self-analysis, you can determine your strengths and weaknesses and, with the help of your instructor, set goals for your physical improvement.

In succeeding chapters guidance is given on how to reach these goals through selected exercises, skilled movement, intelligent use of body levers, health practices, and relaxation. You can design a program of self-improvement to meet your own specific needs and, with hard work and determination, the results will more than repay you for your efforts. But be forewarned before turning the page—all effort will have been in vain if it stops when you reach your goal. It is a sad thought to contemplate, but you will lose that figure/physique and fitness as fast as you gained it, if you do not continue the program. It is a lifetime commitment you are undertaking.

Fitness, Physique and Figure Analysis

Before initiating a program of self-improvement, you need to assess your present status. This chapter describes a battery of tests which measures the health—related aspects of physical fitness: muscular endurance, cardiovascular endurance, strength, flexibility, and body composition. In addition, guidelines are provided for measuring your "shape" (figure/physique). On the basis of the results of these tests and measurements, you should set goals for yourself and design a program of exercises and activities to meet your needs. Subsequent chapters will provide guidance for this purpose.

After taking the tests, record your scores and rankings on Charts I and II in the Appendix. You may wish to repeat the tests periodically to determine whether your program is effective. Chart II should tell you if you are improving, so that you can revise your program if necessary. Those who are enrolled in a formal class may be asked to make a final assessment at the end of the course and record the results on Chart I for comparison with their initial scores.

It is important that you exert maximum effort on each of the performance tests and that you follow the directions for all tests and measures precisely. This will enable you to obtain a true picture of your status and compare your scores with the norms for your age group. Make certain that you warm-up before taking the fitness tests to avoid injury as well as to improve your scores.

Tests for Physical Fitness

Pull-ups (Arm Strength and Endurance). Hang from a bar with palms facing the body. Pull up until the chin is over the bar and then lower the body until the arms are completely extended again. Continue until you can do no more. Do not kick or twist or stay in one position for more than two seconds. Excessive swaying should be prevented by a partner. The score is the total number of pull-ups completed without stopping (up and down = 1 count).

Bent-Arm Hang (For the Person Who Can Not Execute a Pull-up Successfully). Stand on a chair and grasp the bar with palms facing the body. Have someone remove the chair while you hang with your chin over the bar (see illustration) as long as possible, up to 25 seconds. Your score is the number of seconds you were able to hang.

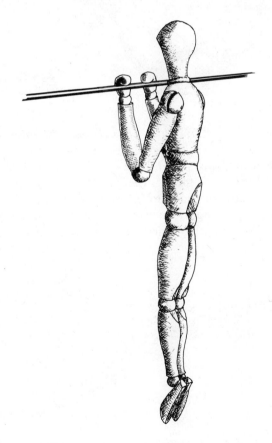

Sit-ups (*Abdominal Strength and Endurance*). Assume a hook-lying position with the fingers clasped behind your neck. An assistant will hold your feet in position. With the knees bent to a 90° angle, flex the spine and roll-up, making at least one elbow touch the knees. You may alternate touching right elbow to left knee and left elbow to right knee or touch both elbows to both knees. On the down movement, the fingers must touch the mat. The score is the total number of correct sit-ups completed in sixty seconds (up and down = 1 count).

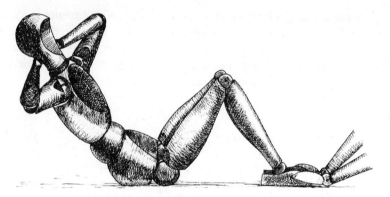

Push-Ups (*Arm and Shoulder Strength and Endurance for Men*). Face the floor and support your body on your toes and hands while keeping the arms and the body straight and stiff. Lower the body by bending the elbows until your nose touches the floor, then push up to the starting position. Do not allow the body to "pike" or "sag" at the hips. Count the number of correct push-ups done continuously (without rest). Down and up = 1 count. You may stop when you can no longer execute a correct push-up.

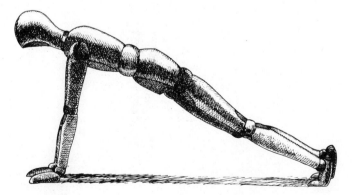

*Modified Push-ups (**Arm and Shoulder Strength and Endurance For Women**).* Assume a modified push-up position with the hands on the floor under the shoulders, arms straight, and knees bent. Keep the body straight from head to knees, while lowering the body until the chest touches the floor. Return to the starting position. Do not allow the hips to bend (pike) or the back to sag (arch). The score is the number of correct push-ups done continuously (down and up = 1 count).

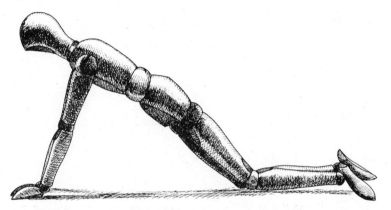

*Sit and Reach (**Flexibility of the Lower Back and Hamstrings**).* Sit on the floor with the legs together and extended, and the soles of the feet against a bench, turned on its side, to which a ruler has been attached. While an assistant holds your knees straight, bounce and reach forward over the ruler three times. Hold the position on the third reach for three seconds minimum. Do *not* touch the ruler during the bounce or the hold. The score is read in inches from the fingertips to the toes (edge of the bench). For example, if you reach to your toes, your score is 0; if you reach six inches past your toes, your score is +6″; if you lack two inches to your toes, your score is —2″.

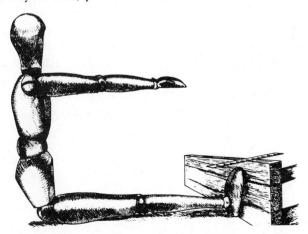

1.5 *Mile Run/Walk* (***Cardiovascular Endurance***). On a measured track, cover the distance of a mile and a half in as short a time as possible. Try to pace yourself so you can jog the entire distance. It is permissable to walk if necessary. On a quarter-mile (one-fourth mile) track, you would run/walk 6 laps while being timed with a stop watch. Your score is the length of time, to the nearest second, in which you covered the distance.

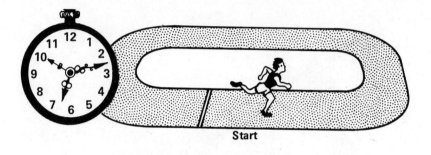

Start

Recording and Interpreting Your Scores

To understand the significance of your scores on the physical fitness tests you may compare your scores with those made by others in the 17-25 age range and with the score you made on another test. For this purpose, Table I presents a set of "norms" with the scores converted to rankings based on the performance of a large number of other young adult men and women.

On Table I, find your score and circle it for each test; then connect the circles with a line to show your profile of physical fitness. Read across the page to find your ranking. If you rank as *excellent,* you are better than 80 percent of college age people; if your score falls in the *good* category, you are better than 60 percent of the population sampled; a rating of *average* means you fall between the 40th and 59th percentile.

A score in the *fair* range means you are below average and a *poor* rating means you are in the lower 20 percent of the young adults sampled. Since these norms are based on college age students from a wide variety of backrounds and fitness levels, being *average* is probably an undesirable goal. You should strive to reach the *good* or *excellent* categories. At the end of the course or at the end of three months, plot your profile with a different colored pencil to observe your improvement.

TABLE I

Physical Fitness Norms for Ages 17-25*

Rank	1.5 mi. run/walk ♂ ♀		sit & reach (both)	Sit-up ♂ ♀		push-ups ♂ ♀		pull-ups ♂ ♀	
	Minutes		Inches						
Excellent	10	13	7.2	44+	34+	45+	31+	15+	3+
Good	11	14	6.4-7.1	39-43	31-44	38-44	26-29	11-14	2
Average	12	15	5.1-6.3	35-38	28-30	32-37	21-25	7-10	1
Fair	13	16	3.9-5.0	30-34	25-27	26-31	14-20	4-6	25 sec.
Poor	14	17	3.8	0-29	0-24	0-25	0-13	3	24 sec. less

* ♂ norms for men; ♀ norms for women; (both) means norms apply to both sexes; pull-up norms for women include bent-arm hang time in the fair and poor category; < means "or less"; > means "or more".

Body Composition

Many people, especially teen agers and young adults, are dissatisfied with their estimated "ideal" weight and feel that they should weigh much less because they want smaller girth measurements. This is usually due to a misconception about body composition and confusion of the terms *weight* and *fatness*. One's fatness is a more important indication of health (and appearance) than one's weight. Most people need to strive for *leanness*, not lightness! It is possible to reduce girth measurements by losing fat and increasing muscle, without changing weight; sometimes one can lose inches and even experience a weight gain!

The percentage of fat in the body can be estimated by several sophisticated laboratory procedures, but one relatively simple method is by skinfold measures. Approximately 50 percent of our total body fat lies just under the skin and can be pinched-up and measured by skin calipers. By measuring several predetermined sites on the body and computing by formulae, a fairly accurate assessment of the relative leanness-fatness composition of the body may be made. This is time consuming and requires considerable experience in the use of calipers; you will need the assistance of an expert. If calipers are available, have a trained person measure you. A simplified version of a skinfold measurement test is to choose one representative site; the midpoint of the back of the upper arm (tricep) provides a reasonably good estimate of fatness.

Refer to Table III to determine whether you are over-fat to the point of being classified as obese. Find your age and sex and read across the page to the measurement. If your own measurement is the same or greater, you are obese. If your measurement is within 2 or 3 millimeter below the score on the table you have too much fat. Read Chapter 2 and Chapter 4 to determine the significance of being over-fat and how to do something about it.

If you have access to the equipment and an expert to measure you, a reasonably accurate assessment of your percentage of body fat can be obtained by summing the measurements from four sites, the triceps, biceps, iliac crest, and scapula. Directions for this are found in the *Instructor's Handbook* which accompanies this text. If this technique or a similar one is used, you should record your scores on Chart II and refer to Table II for your rating.

TABLE II

Fat vs. Lean Rankings

Rank	Men % of Fat	Women % of Fat
Obese	20 or more	28 or more
Over-fat	18 - 19	23 - 27
Average	15 - 17	18 - 22
Lean	11 - 14	16 - 17
Very Lean	10 or less	15 or less

Desirable Body Weight

"Desirable" or "ideal" body weight differs greatly among individuals—even individuals of the same age and height will not necessarily have the same "ideal" weight, because of differences in skeletal size and muscle mass. However, your weight should be within approximately 10 percent of your estimated "ideal" weight. If you are more than ten percent above or below this figure, you may be considered overweight or underweight, respectively. (If you are 20 percent over the "ideal" you are classified as obese.) The "ideal" weight may be modified to some extent by heavy musculature; therefore, an individual may be overweight without being overfat. Some football linemen and weight lifters may be classified as overweight, yet they may not have an ounce of surplus fat on them. On the other hand, some sedentary individuals may be overfat (fat weighs less than muscle) without being overweight. Nevertheless, for all practical purposes, excess weight should be a cause for concern.

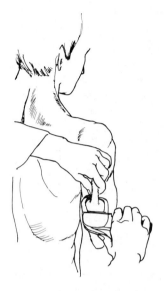

TABLE III

Minimum Triceps Skinfold Thickness
Indicating Obesity*

Age	Males (millimeters)	Females (millimeters)
12	18	22
13	18	23
14	17	23
15	16	24
16	15	25
17	14	26
18	15	27
19	15	27
20	16	28
21	17	28
22	18	28
23	18	28
24	19	28
25	20	29
26	20	29
27	21	29
28	22	29
29	22	29
30-50	23	30

*Adapted from Selzer, C. C. and J. Mayer, "A Simple Criterion of Obesity," *Postgraduate Medicine*, 38 no. 2 (1965), A-101.

Height-Weight Tables are widely used. These are based on average weights of hundreds of individuals of the same height, age, and frame size. The population on which these tables are based does not necessarily represent the general population of the United States, nor do the tables consider the relative amount of fat content; therefore, they should not be considered as totally accurate. To use Table V, it is necessary to determine your frame size. The wrist is a good predictor of the size of one's skeleton. Have a partner measure the wrist by placing the tape above the styloid processes (wrist bones) at the smallest circumference. Record it on Chart I (Appendix) then refer to Table IV to find your approximate skeletal (frame) size. Your height should be measured on a stadiometer, while you are barefooted. Record this on Chart I, also.

TABLE IV

Frame Size Based on Wrist Circumference

	Men	**Women**
Small Frame	6½″ or less	5½″ or less
Medium Frame	6¾″–7¼″	5¾″
Large Frame	7½″ or more	6″ or more

TABLE V-A

"Desirable" Weights for Men*

Height with shoes on (1″ heels) Feet	Inches	Weight in Pounds According to Frame (in Indoor Clothing)		
		Small Frame	Medium Frame	Large Frame
5	2	112-120	118-129	126-141
5	3	115-123	121-133	129-144
5	4	118-126	124-136	132-148
5	5	121-129	127-139	135-152
5	6	124-133	130-143	138-156
5	7	128-137	134-147	142-161
5	8	132-141	138-152	147-166
5	9	136-145	142-156	151-170
5	10	140-150	146-160	155-174
5	11	144-154	150-165	159-179
6	0	148-158	154-170	164-184
6	1	152-162	158-175	168-189
6	2	156-167	162-180	173-194
6	3	160-171	167-185	178-199
6	4	164-175	172-190	182-204

*Used by permission of the Metropolitan Life Insurance Co.

TABLE V-B

Desirable Weights for Women[*]

Height with shoes in (2-inch heels)	Weight in Pounds According to Frame (in Indoor Clothing)		
	Small Frame	Medium Frame	Large Frame
4′10″	92- 98	96-107	104-119
4′11″	94-101	98-110	106-122
5′ 0″	96-104	101-113	109-125
5′ 1″	99-107	104-116	112-128
5′ 2″	102-110	107-119	115-131
5′ 3″	105-113	110-122	118-134
5′ 4″	108-116	113-126	121-138
5′ 5″	111-119	116-130	125-142
5′ 6″	114-123	120-135	129-146
5′ 7″	118-127	124-139	133-150
5′ 8″	122-131	128-143	137-154
5′ 9″	126-135	132-147	141-158
5′10″	130-140	136-151	145-163
5′11″	134-144	140-155	149-168
6′ 0″	138-148	144-159	153-173

[*]Used by permission of Metropolitan Life Insurance Company.

If you are weighing in a leotard or gym suit, you will weigh one or two pounds lighter than you would in "street clothes". If you weigh in shoes, you will weigh a pound or two more than the chart allows for. To read Table V-A or V-B, find your height (with shoes) in the left column for the Table appropriate to your sex; then with a straight edge, read directly across to the column which is appropriate for your frame size. Record your "ideal weight" on Chart I (Appendix). Note: If you measured your height while *barefooted*, to interpret the Table, use the height on the Table which is one-inch taller than your measured height.

Ideal Measurements

It is difficult to define what we mean by ideal measurements when referring to the figure. At one time in history, Venus De Milo, with her forty-three-inch bust, thirty-eight-inch waist and forty-four-inch hips, was considered the perfect female figure. Very few women today feel that these measurements are ideal; neither do most men accept the 18″ neck, 54″ chest and 19″ arm of a "Mr. Universe" as a perfect physique for them. Fashions and fads have much to do with what we consider ideal.

Body build influences your measurements. A person with a large bony structure naturally has larger measurements than a person with small bones, yet each measurement can be considered ideal for that individual. There are three basic types of body builds that we may inherit. These are classified according to linearity, muscularity, and fat distribution. The *ectomorph* is slender, characterized by having a large forehead, small bones, a long, slender neck, slender arms and legs, a narrow chest, round shoulders with winged scapulae, a flat abdomen, and inconspicuous buttocks. The *mesomorph* has firm muscles and large bones, and is ruggedly built with prominent facial bones, a rather long, muscular neck, wide, sloping shoulders, a broad chest, muscular arms, a heavily muscled abdomen, a low waist, narrow hips, muscular buttocks, and powerful legs. The *endomorph* is round and soft and characterized by having a round head, a short neck, narrow shoulders, fatty breasts and abdomen, short arms, wide hips, heavy buttocks, and short, heavy legs. Few people have a build which perfectly fits one of these types. More than likely you are a combination type, such as an ecto-mesomorph or a meso-endomorph.

Because of hereditary differences in our body build, it is not realistic to expect the majority of the population to have the same body proportions. However, because of a national preoccupation with body measurements, the following guidelines are offered, based on the measurements of thousands of men and women who are considered well proportioned.

TABLE VI

Body Proportion Guidelines*

	Men	**Women**
Chest/Bust	Same as hip	(see hip)
Waist	5-7″ less than chest or hip	8-10″ smaller than bust
Abdomen	1 1/2-2 1/2″ smaller than chest	1 1/2-2 1/2″ smaller than bust
Hips	Same as chest	same as bust if slim hips 1-3″ larger than bust for av. hips 3-4″ larger than bust for full hips
Thighs	8-10″ less than waist	6-7″ less than waist
Calves	7-8″ less than thigh	6-7″ less than thigh
Ankles	6-7″ less than calves	5-6″ less than calves
Upper Arm	Twice the circumference of the wrist	twice the circumference of the wrist

*From *The West Point Fitness and Diet Book,* by Colonel James L. Anderson and Martin Cohen. Copyright © 1977 by Colonel James L. Anderson and Martin Cohen. Reprinted by permission of Rawson, Wade Publishers.

How to Measure

Record your measurements on Charts I and II in the Appendix, along with the goals you are striving to achieve. Measurements should be taken by a partner because you cannot measure yourself accurately. Stand relaxed with your weight evenly distributed on both feet, arms at sides. Do not suck-in your waist or contract muscles to alter your measurements. The tape measure should be kept parallel to the floor and pulled snugly but not tight enough to indent the skin. You should wear as little clothing as possible (underwear, bathing suit or leotards), and when you are measured at later dates, make certain that you are dressed in the same manner. It is also advisable always to measure at the same time of day if an accurate record of progress is to be kept. Do not measure after exercise, since the muscles will be temporarily enlarged. Measure to the nearest eighth of an inch (or centimeter if the metric scale is used).

Bust—Partner should stand and measure from the front at the largest girth (nipple line) at the mid-point of a normal breath.

Waist—Partner should stand and measure from the front at the smallest girth between the ribs and the crest of the iiium.

Abdomen—Partner should kneel and measure from the side at the largest girth between waist and hips, usually just below the navel.

Hips—Partner should kneel and measure from the side at the largest girth, approximately level with the pubic bone.

Thigh—Partner should kneel in front and measure upper thigh of the dominant leg* at the largest girth, usually an inch or two below the crotch and directly under buttocks.

Calf—Partner should kneel at the side and measure the largest girth of the dominant leg* usually about two-thirds of the way up from the ankle.

Ankle—Partner should kneel at the side and measure the smallest girth of the dominant leg just above the ankle bones.

Upper Arm—Partner should stand at the side and measure over the largest part of the bicep, midway between the shoulder and elbow. The subject should raise the dominant arm, palm up parallel to floor. The tape should be perpendicular to the floor. The arm should remain relaxed.

*Dominant leg is the leg you would normally use to kick a ball.

Fitness and Exercise

2

In the last half of the twentieth century there has been a growing interest in the physical aspects of good health and physical fitness. Beginning with Eisenhower in 1956, the last seven presidents of the United States have deemed physical fitness sufficiently important to appoint a President's Council on Physical Fitness and Sports. Leading national organizations such as the American Alliance for Health, Physical Education, Recreation and Dance, the American Heart Association, the American Medical Association, and the Public Health Service, have encouraged and supported the principle that individuals should have a healthy life style which includes being physically fit. Physical fitness is not a cure-all, but by combining it with proper diet, rest and relaxation, abstention from smoking, abstention or moderation in alcohol and drug usage, and wise management of stress, you will add years to your life and life to your years.

Positive Health Concepts

Good health is a possession to be valued highly, but most individuals are not concerned with maintaining or improving it until it is seriously threatened. It is something you cannot buy in a drugstore or health food store, nor can it be given to you. You have to work to achieve this aspect of the "good life;" you have to do it yourself. The positive qualities to strive for are:

1. A high energy level developed through improved physical fitness, particularly of the cardiovascular and respiratory systems (achieved by exercising vigorously).
2. Optimal muscle strength, endurance, and mobility (achieved by exercising vigorously).
3. Optimal nutrition (achieved by consuming the right foods in the right amounts).

4. An ideal body composition—a lean body with a low percentage of fat (achieved by observing nos. 1, 2 and 3 above).
5. The ability to relax and sleep; (aided by a vigorous life style, regular habits of rest, and the use of relaxation techniques).
6. A happy disposition and excellent mental health (achieved through continuing emotional growth).
7. A well integrated personality (resulting from the first 6).[1]

The level of health you can achieve is determined largely by heredity; but there are other contributing factors over which you have little or no control, including accidents, certain diseases or conditions, and aging. The extent to which you develop your health potential depends upon your life style. It is worth the effort to make changes in your living patterns in order to develop these positive health qualities. Being "healthy" means that you can get through the stresses of the day and still have the energy and desire to be active in leisure pursuits. It can be the difference between attending or cutting classes, being safe or having an accident, being comfortable or aching, enjoying or loathing an activity. With good health you will be able to live more effectively within your capabilities—now is the time to begin to improve your life style.

Physical Fitness Defined

Physical fitness, a quality of positive health, is specific to each individual. It is the "physical condition" that allows you to do your work efficiently and effectively, pursue leisure time activities vigorously and alertly, and respond to emergencies successfully during an ordinary day. There is a difference of opinion as to what components constitute physical fitness, because some authors list only health related components while others expand the list to include skill-related factors such as agility, power, speed, balance, reaction time, and coordination. Skill related fitness is important, but this text limits discussion to the five basic components of health related fitness—strength, muscular endurance, cardiovascular endurance, flexibility, and body composition.

- Strength is measured by the amount of force a muscle can exert against resistance in one effort, or, for example, how much weight can be lifted.
- Muscular endurance may be defined as the ability of a muscle to apply force repeatedly, or to sustain a contraction for a long period of time. The longer it can contract without tiring, the better its endurance.

- Cardiovascular endurance, (sometimes referred to as cardiorespiratory) is a measure of the ability of the heart and lungs to provide fuel to the tissues and carry off waste products during sustained exercise. It is commonly referred to as one's "wind." A typical test of this type of endurance is to run for as long as possible. The sooner you become winded and the longer it takes you to recover "your breath" and resting heart rate, the poorer your cardiovascular endurance.

- Flexibility is a measure of the range of motion in the joints of the body. The length of the muscles, tendons, and ligaments largely determines how much freedom of motion one has. Stretching exercises are used to increase flexibility. For example, your ability to assume a long sitting position and touch your toes without bending your knees is a measure of the flexibility in your lower back and posterior leg muscles.

- Body composition is the relative percentage of fat and lean (fat free) body mass. Having too much fat makes the circulatory system work harder and places stress on all body systems. Excessive fatness is associated with coronary heart disease, high blood pressure, diabetes, and other health problems.

Why Exercise?

As we entered the decade of the 1980s automation continued to escalate; the aim of modern technology seems to be to eliminate human physical effort. The habit of physical activity in our daily lives is being lost—we ride to classes, put motors on our bicycles, push buttons to have machines do our work, and watch sporting events in the arenas and on television rather than taking an active part. In 1910 people had a six-day, 72 hour work week. Seventy years later most people worked a 40 hour week spread over five days, with some condensing their work time into four days. In the future we expect to work even fewer days and less hours. This means more and more leisure time to be used wisely or not so wisely.

What is happening to our health status? There are some positive gains to report. Surveys show that the mortality rate from heart ailments declined by more than 30 percent in the last 30 years and that two years were added to our normal life expectancy.[2] However, it is obvious that many Americans do not live wisely. Too many are overweight; according to the Metropolitan Life Insurance Company, nearly 37 million women and 33 million men are 10 percent or more overweight.[3] Cardiovascular disease, frequently attributed to obesity and physical inactivity, remains the primary killer. As many as 75 million Americans have back problems (often associated with poor body mechanics and physical inactivity); beyond the personal pain of backache, there is a financial impact of 93 million work days lost each year.[4]

Organically, humans are active creatures—they are not meant to lead sedentary lives. We possess the capacities for movement and the neuromuscular mechanism to produce it. Our growth and development depend upon physical activity. According to the "law of use and disuse," without activity, atrophy (wasting away) of size and function sets in and experiences become limited.

Your body has 206 bones and 639 muscles. The muscles are made up of uncounted millions of muscle fibers. Each fiber possesses a slender nerve strand which fires up to 75 impulses per second. There are thousands of miles of nerves and thousands of nerve centers which determine your movements, thoughts, memories, and imagination. Your heart pumps thirteen tons of blood per day (you have 5 to 6 quarts of blood) through 100,000 miles of blood vessels. To keep this complex mechanism in working order, exercise, which contributes to total fitness, is essential.

Exercise is an integral part of normal human life. Physical activity is necessary to the maintenance of physical and emotional health. While you are in school, it is usually easy to find time and space to exercise, since the facilities and opportunities are available. After graduation, many people stop exercising regularly because gymnasiums are not as accessible, interests change, while demands of job and home crowd out recreational pursuits. As a result, the adult must make an extra effort to keep exercise in the daily routine, since the need continues throughout life. Therefore, plan and prepare now to make wise use of your leisure time today, tomorrow, and in years to come.

Immediate Effects of Exercise

The effects of physical activity upon the tissues and functions of the body depend upon a number of factors. Very light exercise, continued for a short period of time, produces negligible effect upon the body. Fairly strenuous activity, continued for a reasonable period of time, has certain immediate effects on the body. These may be stated briefly as follows:

1. The heart beats faster; the blood and lymph circulate faster through the body tissues. The effect of the increased blood supply is to bring greater amounts of food and oxygen to the body cells and carry away waste products of cellular activity more rapidly.

2. Breathing becomes deeper and is more frequent. This acceleration is necessary in order to supply the greater amount of oxygen necessary to provide energy and to remove waste products.
3. A greater number of red corpuscles appear in the blood stream, making it possible for more oxygen to be carried to the body tissues.
4. The body temperature rises, resulting in sweating to dissipate heat through the skin.
5. The metabolic rate increases as more food is utilized to supply necessary energy and it becomes necessary to remove more waste products.
6. The working muscles increase in volume due to the increased blood flow.
7. Arteries supplying the active muscles become more dilated and the blood vessels in the inactive areas become more constricted. This allows the blood to go to the area where it is most needed.
8. Most of the body cells are stimulated through the increased blood and lymph supplies.

When one engages regularly in a moderate amount of invigorating physical activity the mechanisms of respiration, circulation, and elimination become increasingly more efficient in their functions of supplying food and oxygen to working cells and eliminating waste products. Regular exercise of reasonable intensity and duration, then, vitalizes and invigorates the body tissues, raising their efficiency to a higher level. Lack of exercise tends to cause tissues to become inefficient in performing their functions.

Long Range Health Benefits of Regular Exercise

Most medical and health leaders agree that exercise is important for everyone. The benefits you receive will depend upon your age, present fitness level, and the type, level of intensity, duration, and frequency of the activity. Research has proved the following long range benefits of regular exercise:

1. The aging process is delayed.
2. Life expectancy is increased.
3. The possibility or severity of several diseases or conditions is reduced including:

   a. Coronary heart disease   f. Osteoporosis
   b. Hypertension   g. Backache
   c. Obesity   h. Diabetes mellitus
   d. Arteriosclerosis   i. Chronic lung disease
   e. Angina   j. Asthma

4. Physical fitness is improved (increased strength, endurance, flexibility, and leanness).
5. Minor aches and pains, stiffness, and soreness are less frequent.
6. Remediable postural defects are improved.
7. General appearance is improved.
8. Efficiency is increased and the expenditure of energy in performing both physical and mental tasks is reduced.
9. Tension is reduced and ability to relax is improved.
10. Chronic fatique is reduced.
11. Recovery in hospitals is faster when early ambulation is instituted.

Anatomical and Physiological Changes

The benefits listed above are in large part due to several anatomical and physiological changes which accompany improvement in strength, endurance, and flexibility. These are summarized as follows:

1. The heart size increases, resulting in greater stroke volume and more cardiac output, which in turn cause a lower resting heart rate and a smaller increase in heart rate for a given increase in work.
2. The blood volume increases and there is a change in the composition—more red blood corpuscles and less water content increase its oxygen carrying capacity.
3. The number of capillaries increases, resulting in increased vascularization. (This is particularly important for the heart muscle.)
4. The interior volume of the lungs increases, allowing a larger exchange of air per breath. This results in a decreased respiratory rate during rest and a smaller increase in the rate during heavy work.
5. The number of active muscle fibers increases, as well as the size of the muscle fibers, resulting in an increase in the size of the muscle.
6. There is an increase in muscle strength and improved neural functioning.
7. There is an increase in neuromuscular efficiency due to:
   a. the reduction of fatty tissues in the muscles;
   b. the decreased resistance from antagonistic muscles;
   c. more efficient transmission of nerve impulses;
   d. less wasted motion;
   e. improved efficiency in the contractile processes of the muscle fibers.

Points to Consider Before
Beginning Your Exercise Program

Exercises are not a panacea. The information in this chapter is to assist you in selecting the activity and the amount necessary to develop and/or maintain your desired or acceptable level of fitness, and to improve your health status and personal appearance. Prior to planning your exercise regimen there are several points to be considered.

1. The time of day is not important except that it must fit into your schedule. The least desirable time would be immediately after a meal, when strenuous exertion might make you uncomfortable.

2. Muscle soreness, characterized by generalized pain and stiffness upon movement, is a natural result of exercise when you are unaccustomed to the activity. Repeating the activity the next day is the best cure for soreness.

3. Be realistic in your goals, and do not expect changes overnight. You did not get in your present "shape" overnight!

4. Women do not need to worry about developing bulging muscles— it is highly improbable. Just remember that firm muscles are more attractive than sagging ones.

5. Exercise, combined with a reduction in caloric intake, is by far the most satisfactory method of losing weight.

6. Avoid taking your measurements immediately after exercise, because muscles tend to hypertrophy (increase in size) during and immediately after exercise.

7. Exercises do not insure good posture; however, they do make it easier to attain and maintain.

8. If you are trying to lose weight, do not worry about increasing your appetite as a result of exercise. Studies show that it is negligible and that you will burn more calories than you will take in.

9. The average woman is able to participate in most activities during her menstrual period. Lack of sufficient exercise is often a cause of dysmenorrhea, and some exercise can actually give relief from menstrual cramps.

10. After childhood, muscular activity does not affect the bony structure. Do not expect to attain trim ankles if the cause of the size of your ankles is large bone structure. Exercise will not change the size of the bone.

11. Heredity is the major factor in determining the size of a woman's bust (breasts). Exercises will develop chest muscles, and when combined with good posture this can enhance your figure or physique.

12. Endurance activities which require running and jumping generally cause more debilitating injuries to beginning exercisers than other non-weight bearing activities.
13. In order to maintain the training effect, exercise must be continued on a regular basis, or you will return to near pretraining levels of fitness.
14. There is no such thing as "effortless exercise." Fancy machines, girdles, belts, and couches are not effective for "spot reducing," "breaking up fatty deposits," or "melting away fat"—they only melt away your purse!

General Suggestions for Exercising

In order to gain the maximum benefit and enjoyment from an exercise program (for conditioning and/or reducing), and at the same time to suffer a minimum of discomfort, you will find the following suggestions useful:

1. Have a thorough medical examination and the approval of your physician before participating.
2. Seek the advice of your physician if you have a serious illness, operation or injury after you have started your program. No one else (including physical educators) is qualified to determine the type and amount of exercise that is advisable.
3. Dress appropriately so that you can move freely and safely; this includes footwear as well as clothes.
4. Perform exercise regularly—three to five times per week.
5. Exercise in the target zone for each fitness component.
6. Plan a definite time for your workouts and adhere to it—preferably the same time each day. Exercise should become as much a part of your daily routine as bathing and dressing.
7. Find a comfortable position to begin an exercise, and stabilize other body parts to prevent muscle strain. Use padding to avoid pressure on bony areas which might become bruised and tender.
8. Start the exercise gradually—begin with a minimum number and increase the number of repetitions gradually over a period of time until you reach your goal. The gradual approach will help to avoid soreness and muscle strain.
9. Do not overdo it. You should be able to repeat the exercises the next day without undue soreness or stiffness.
10. Be aware of signs of overexertion—severe breathlessness, dizziness, tightness or pain in your chest, loss of muscle control, and nausea. If you experience any of these, stop immediately.

11. Perform the exercise slowly (with no quick, jerky motions) to help prevent soreness and to alleviate it.
12. Take particular care in doing abdominal exercises. Initially, choose mild exercises and do only a few of these—gradually increasing the number of exercises and their severity. Do not develop the familiar muscle soreness in this area.
13. Start each exercise period with light exercises (preferably flexibility exercises) to warm-up; then gradually work into more vigorous exercises. Flexibility exercises performed prior to more strenuous ones tend to reduce the risk of muscle, tendon, and ligament injuries.
14. Breathe normally during the performance of the exercise unless the instructions specifically state that you do otherwise. If you will inhale during the recovery phase and exhale on the effort phase, the exercise may seem easier.
15. Emphasize proper technique and full range of motion. Exercise slowly and rhythmically, concentrating on strong muscular effort.
16. Include activities for most of the large muscle groups. Do not spend an activity period working on one set of muscles alone.
17. Pay attention to weak areas and do not perform only the exercises you like.
18. Maintain the fun element; the exercise period can leave you refreshed in mind and body. If it becomes a drudgery, add a variety of exercises, companionship, musical accompaniment, or change in scenery.
19. Keep the exercise period relatively short (20-40 minutes) and well organized to avoid boredom and discouragement. Strength and endurance exercises might be performed Mondays, Wednesdays, Fridays, and aerobic activities Tuesdays, Thursdays, Saturdays, while flexibility exercises are included in every workout.
20. Avoid dehydration; drink liquids when you are thirsty. Water is an excellent fluid replacement.
21. Start each exercise period with a warm-up and end with a cool-down. A nice warm shower or bath will complete that feeling of "relaxed well-being."

Exercises for Figure/Physique Improvement

Physical fitness, posture, figure/physique, and weight control are interrelated and overlapping. The same exercises can be used for all these purposes. And, believe it or not, the same exercise which helps the flabby person *decrease* measurements may help the thin person *increase* measurements.

Both localized exercises (those for specific areas such as push-ups for the upper trunk and arms), and general exercises (such as jogging and swimming) are effective in "taking off inches." We suggest you do both to insure that all muscle groups receive maximum benefit. Also, we strongly urge you to participate in dance and sports; their psychological value will complement their sociological and psychological benefits.

When designing a program to "shape-up," choose specific calisthenics for selected body regions you want to improve. Generally, it will be to your advantage to combine these with weight training and aerobic exercises. Men probably will benefit more from weight training exercises if they desire changes in physique, since calisthenics might not produce an overload to bring about strengthening with accompanying muscle bulge.

Finally. remember that weight and figure/physique are not synomymous. If you consider yourself too broad in the hips or fat around the middle, this doesn't necessarily mean that you need to lose weight. If your weight approaches normalcy, your problem may be flabbiness or fat—not weight.

Questionable Exercises

Not all exercises are good, nor are good exercises beneficial for all. Many popular magazines and television shows (even some professional literature) advocate exercises which could be harmful. They may also claim certain exercises to be beneficial to specific muscle groups which in reality are not involved. The following are some examples of such practices and some cautions to be observed.

Questionable Abdominal Exercises

Double Leg Lifts. Raising and lowering straight legs from a back-lying position is a dangerous exercise because it puts great strain on the lower back and may stretch or even rupture the abdominal muscles. This is not an abdominal-strengthening exercise, because the abdominal muscles are not attached to the legs. The muscles used are the hip flexors. If you had strong enough abdominal muscles to keep your back from arching during this exercise, it probably would not be harmful—but then, you would not need the exercise.

Sit-ups with Legs Straight. Like the double leg lift, this sit-up exercise uses the hip flexor muscles rather than the abdominals and may result in the same undesirable arched back and stretched abdominals. If it was executed so that the pelvis was tilted backward, and the lower back remained in contact with the floor while the spine curled up, it probably would not be harmful.

The safest, most effective abdominal strengthening exercises are trunk curls or isometric exercises. When adequate strength has been developed, sit-ups with bent knees might be attempted—but remember to curl up and keep your lower back flat. More advanced sit-ups can be done by changing the arm position, using a tilt board, or adding weights.

Questionable Back Exercises

If you have lordosis (swayback), weak abdominals, or back problems, you should avoid exercises which allow the pelvis to tilt forward to stretch the abdominal muscles or arch the back. Such exercises as back bends, prone arm and leg lifts (swan position), and backward circling of the trunk are not advised.

Questionable Shoulder Exercises

It has been estimated that 80 percent of the students have round shoulders; therefore, exercises which promote this condition should be avoided. Such things as push-ups, chinning, and forward-arm circling strengthen and shorten the already shortened pectoral (chest) muscles and should be avoided, *unless* they are balanced by activities which will stretch those muscles and strengthen the upper back and posterior shoulder muscles.

Questionable Leg Exercises

Deep knee bends may damage the knee joint by pinching the synovial membrane, which provides lubrication of the joint, or by stretching the knee ligaments. Exercises which cause the knee to bend more than 90° such as the duck walk, Russian bear dance, and squat thrust are among those which should be avoided. Half knee bends (90° knee flexion) are acceptable, but the feet should always be directly under the knees to prevent a twist of the joint.

Doing, or attempting to do, the "splits" can cause serious damage. Most individuals are not anatomically built to assume this position, nor do they have a need to be so flexible in this area.

Rising on the toes and maintaining this position strengthens and shortens the "calf" but stretches the plantar structures of the feet and weakens the arch. Part of the stretching can be eliminated by keeping the feet inverted (point toes in) when you stand on your tiptoes. Exercises which dorsiflex the foot (bring the toes toward the knee) should be used to help maintain muscular balance and keep the calf from becoming too tight.

Questionable Flexibility Exercises

This subject is a controversial one, but since it probably is better to err on the side of caution, it is mentioned here. Some people frown on the practice of stretching the hamstrings (posterior leg muscles) and lower back muscles by doing a standing toe-touch exercise. The usual method is to stand with straight legs, and try to touch the floor or toes by bouncing. It is felt that this exercise might lead to back strain and sciatica (because the sciatic nerve is stretched).

The same exercise, done in a long-sitting position, would be less apt to damage structures because the body attains less momentum in the absence of gravity; therefore, the stretching force is less strenuous.

Frequently one hears or reads that toe touching is a good abdominal exercise. This is not true. It is a flexibility exercise and will not strengthen the abdominal muscles.

Principles of Exercise

You will not develop an adequate level of physical fitness immediately. It will take time and effort; (how much depends upon your present status and the type of exercise you are doing) to achieve a level that will meet your current and or anticipated needs. The program, directed toward the improvement of the five fitness components, should be individually and systematically designed with you in mind. You must participate regularly, at least three times a week, and follow the basic physiological principles of overload and adaptation, progression, and specificity.

Overload and Adaptation

Your body systems tend to adapt to your daily routine—they become conditioned to meet these demands and no more. To improve this condition *make the systems (such as the heart, lungs, and muscles) "work" beyond the daily demand so that the amount of work being done is near maximum.* When you have adapted yourself to this new work level, increase the load until eventually your desired working level is reached. The overload (load beyond previous requirements) can be in the form of added weight or resistance, more repetitions, longer work periods, or a greater range of motion. It depends upon which of the five fitness components is being developed. There is a target zone of intensity, duration, and frequency which is optimum for each individual for each component of fitness. If you exercise below the threshold level, no change will occur. Likewise, exercising beyond the upper limits of the target zone will not bring good results because of injury and fatigue factors.

Progression

Although the overload and adaptation principle is used to bring about changes in your body, you must gradually progress from what is considered to be a light work load for you to a heavy one. It is necessary to measure your current fitness status, since the beginning work load should be based upon this. Continue to measure your progress regularly in order to gradually increase your work load as the body adapts to each new change. A systematic program of gradually increasing the exercise difficulty will help prevent injuries, muscle soreness, and discouragement. You cannot become fit overnight. It will require four to six weeks of work before marked improvement is achieved.

Specificity

When exercise is specific, it will develop only that fitness component it is designed to develop and only the body part that is being used. Weight training exercises are not designed to develop flexibility nor is jogging designed to develop arm strength. Select exercises to involve the specific areas you want to change. If you want to build strength, do heavy resistance work; if you want to improve your cardiovascular endurance, involve large muscle groups to bring about an increased heart rate for extended periods of time; if you want to develop flexibility in your lower back, perform exercises that stretch these muscles.

Types of Contractions

Muscles contract in these ways: they may shorten, with the ends being brought toward the center (*concentric*): they may lengthen, with the ends moving away from the center (*eccentric*): or they may hold, without changing length. For example, when doing a push-up exercise the movement upward is a concentric contraction; the movement downward is an eccentric contraction. Contractions involving changes in muscle length (concentric and eccentric) are referred to as isotonic or dynamic contractions. Those involving no change in muscle length (a held contraction) are referred to as isometric or static contractions. For example, in the push-up exercise if you pause on the upward movement and hold the body in the mid position for a few seconds, the muscles will be contracting isometrically. All types of contractions can develop strength and muscular endurance, but only the isotonic type can improve cardiovascular endurance and flexibility.

Training Effect

You can achieve a desirable level of physical fitness by selecting exercises with your particular goals in mind, then setting up a program, and following the general suggestions for exercising (see Chapter 3). The length of time it will take for you to reach your goals will depend upon your age and present level of physical condition. After you have reached your goals, your "training" should not end: a physical-maintenance program should be followed to keep you at this desired level.

Strength

This component of fitness can be developed by using isotonic exercises, isometric exercises, or a combination of the two forms; but you must overload the muscles in the target zone and increase the load progressively. Your muscles should contract against a heavy resistance at regular intervals (three days per week) to the point of maximum exertion. This resistance may be found in your work (e.g. lifting heavy objects), in your athletic endeavors (e.g. breaking a wrestling hold), calisthenics (e.g. lifting your body weight), weight training exercises, or exercises involving applying force against an immovable object (e.g. pushing against a wall or another part of the body).

Three to five isometric contractions of six to eight seconds against maximum resistance, followed by relaxation, will develop strength. Strength may also be developed by isotonic exercises, lifting 75 percent of the maximum weight you can lift in one effort, in three sets of four to eight repetitions. (See Chapter 3 for details on training methods and exercises.)

Muscular Endurance

This second component of fitness is helped somewhat by muscular strength because if you are strong, you may be able to continue exercise for extended periods of time. However, strength and endurance are not the same. If you want to develop endurance, you should work against light to moderate resistance, doing a large number (20 to 30) of repetitions. Progressively overloading the muscles either in weight or repetitions can be done by weight training or by calisthenics; other activities such as jogging, jumping rope, and bicycling can be used for leg muscle endurance.

Cardiovascular Endurance

This fitness component is developed by performing activities which apply stress to the heart as well as to the circulatory and respiratory systems. They should be maintained continuously and rhythmically, and be aerobic (with oxygen) in nature. Examples of suitable activities are full court basketball, racquetball, swimming, jogging, and bicycling. They must be performed regularly (three to five days per week), with intensity (generally 60 percent to 90 percent for the young, healthy individual), and for appropriate periods of time (15 to 60 minutes). The interrelation among frequency, intensity, and duration makes it possible to be flexible in setting up an exercise program.

For example, you would need to work for about 45 minutes (duration) at about 40 percent of your maximum heart rate (intensity) to achieve the same results as exercising for about 15 minutes at a 60 percent working capacity. Exercise periods with the higher heart rates are for the young and healthy adults; work periods with lower heart rates are more realistic for those who are older or who have a low level of fitness.

One method of calculating the intensity needed to put your workout in the target zone is described here. (A worksheet is found in the Appendix, Chart III.) First determine your resting heart rate (RHR), that is, the number of heart beats per minute while you are sitting. Then, establish your maximum heart rate (MHR) by subtracting your age from 220. For example, twenty-year old Sammy has a maximum heart rate of 200 (220-20). If her resting heart rate is 72, she can find her estimated work capacity by subtracting the RHR from the MHR. If she chooses to work at 60 percent of her capacity, she will multiply the difference by .60 and then add her RHR. (see sample)

$$
\begin{array}{rl}
& 220 \\
- & \underline{20} \quad \text{(Age)} \\
& 200 \quad \text{(MHR)} \\
- & \underline{72} \quad \text{(RHR)} \\
& 128 \quad \text{(Estimated working capacity or heart rate range—HRR)} \\
\times & \underline{.60} \quad \text{(percent of working capacity)} \\
& 76.80 \\
+ & \underline{72.00} \quad \text{(RHR)} \\
& 148.8 \text{ or } 149 \text{ beats per minute (work intensity needed for aerobic} \\
& \qquad \text{fitness)}
\end{array}
$$

Flexibility

The fourth fitness component is developed and maintained by regularly moving body parts through a full range of motion, thus stretching the muscle and connective tissue that surround the joint(s). You can exercise alone or have a partner assist you. Either *ballistic* (momentum produced by bobbing or bouncing) or *static* (contracting muscles and holding a position or having a partner move the body segment) forms of stretching exercises can make you more flexible. Exercises that are performed more slowly (static stretch) are less likely to result in injuries or soreness than those executed with the bobbing ((ballistic) movement; however, both types can be beneficial. The method you choose depends upon your condition and your reason for doing the exercise. For best results:

1. Perform the exercises daily
2. Apply the three principles of exercise—overload and adaptation, specificity, and progression
3. Do not overstretch by forcing the movement to the point of pain
4. Hold the static stretch in the extended position for 20 to 30 seconds
5. Perform the ballistic stretch gently and only after preceding it with static stretch and only on healthy joints where there is no history of previous injuries.

Body Composition

Women possess more fat relative to body weight than men; however, their bodies react to physical activity and diet (the means to alter body composition) in the same ways. Either generalized aerobic or localized calisthenic-type exercise is effective in decreasing body fat while adding lean body weight. Performing aerobic activities such as jogging, swimming, jumping rope and climbing stairs at least three days a week for 30 minute sessions at a work capacity of 140-150 bpm (heart rate) for eight weeks should result in significant changes in body composition. The localized exercise such as bent knee sit-ups, push-ups, side leg-raises and side stretchers can be equally effective provided it is performed for the same length of time at the same level of intensity (140-150 bpm). See Chapter 4 for information concerning the diet.

References

1. Herbert A. DeVries, *Health Science: A Positive Approach* (Santa Monica, Ca.: Goodyear Publishing Company, Inc., 1979).
2. "The Fitness Mania," *U.S. News & World Report* (February 27, 1978), 37-40.
3. *Ibid.*
4. "That Aching Back," *Time* (July 14, 1980), 30-38.

Exercises for Fitness, Figure, and Physique

3

During the 1970s Americans appeared to "discover" physical activity. Millions walked, jogged, swam, cycled, played sports, fenced, and did calisthenics. A 1978 report revealed that almost one-half of Americans, age 20 or older, stated that they exercised on a regular basis.[1]

Many individuals choose to participate in exercise activities, rather than sports activities, because being an "athlete" is not a prerequisite, the dollar cost can be minimal, and one can either work alone or with others. Also exercises can be more easily adjusted to the environment (primarily time and space factors) and designed to meet specific needs and interests. There are numerous exercise programs available which have been designed by experts. You may want to use them as guides to design a program for yourself keeping in mind the principles of overload and adaptation, specificity, and progression. The programs in this Chapter are a few of the more popular ones.

Cardiovascular Fitness

Aerobic Exercises

Aerobic means "with oxygen." Included in this category are those exercises which place a strenuous demand on the cardiovascular and respiratory systems (heart, blood vessels, and lungs). These exercises should be done at the target heart rate for 15 to 30 minutes. Young adults usually have a target zone of between 135 to 160 beats per minute. The more intense the exercise the less time is needed but it should not be less than 15 minutes, three days per week. Exercises such as running, jogging, swimming, and bicycling are used widely by people of all ages. Activities such as handball, squash, basketball, team handball, and rope jumping can be used also.

It would be helpful in planning a program to know your present level of aerobic fitness. One test that you can use is the *12-minute run*. See how much distance you can cover with 12 minutes of running, jogging, and/or walking. Check Table VII to find your fitness category. Another test that you can take is the *1½-mile run*. This is discussed in Chapter 1.

TABLE VII
12-Minute Walking/Running Test*
Distance (Miles) Covered in 12 Minutes

FITNESS CATEGORY		AGE (Years)					
		13-19	20-29	30-39	40-49	50-59	60 +
I. Very poor	(men)	<1.30**	<1.22	<1.18	<1.14	<1.03	<.87
	(women)	<1.0	<.96	<.94	<.88	<.84	<.78
II. Poor	(men)	1.30-1.37	1.22-1.31	1.18-1.30	1.14-1.24	1.03-1.16	.87-1.02
	(women)	1.00-1.18	.96-1.11	.95-1.05	.88-.98	.84-.93	.78-.86
III. Fair	(men)	1.38-1.56	1.32-1.49	1.31-1.45	1.25-1.39	1.17-1.30	1.03-1.20
	(women)	1.19-1.29	1.12-1.22	1.06-1.18	.99-1.11	.94-1.05	.87-.98
IV. Good	(men)	1.57-1.72	1.50-1.64	1.46-1.56	1.40-1.53	1.31-1.44	1.21-1.32
	(women)	1.30-1.43	1.23-1.34	1.19-1.29	1.12-1.24	1.06-1.18	.99-1.09
V. Excellent	(men)	1.73-1.86	1.65-1.76	1.57-1.69	1.54-1.65	1.45-1.58	1.33-1.55
	(women)	1.44-1.51	1.35-1.45	1.30-1.39	1.25-1.34	1.19-1.30	1.10-1.18
VI. Superior	(men)	>1.87	>1.77	>1.70	>1.66	>1.59	>1.56
	(women)	>1.52	>1.46	>1.40	>1.35	>1.31	>1.19

*From The Aerobics Way by Kenneth H. Cooper, M.D., M. P.H. Copyright © 1977 by Kenneth H. Cooper. Reprinted by permission or the publishers, M. Evans & Co., Inc., New York 10017.

** < Means "less than"; > means "more than."

Pulse Rated Programs. To develop aerobic power the healthy young adult should train by performing the activity at about 60 percent working capacity. Select an activity which elevates your pulse rate to 135 to 160 beats per minute and sustain the activity at that level of intensity for 20 minutes. If you are a habitually sedentary individual, a pulse rate of 110 to 120 beats per minute may be of suitable intensity at the beginning.

To check to see if you are going too fast too soon, count your pulse five minutes after you have stopped the activity. If the rate is over 120 beats per minute, you need to perform at a lower level. At the end of 10 minutes the rate should be below 100. Another tell-tale sign is your breathing rate. If you are still having difficulty breathing 10 minutes after ending the activity, you are performing at a level too high for you.

Running programs are frequently used to develop cardiovascular fitness. As with any exercise program you should warm-up and cool down slowly; include stretching exercises for the arms, legs, and back. Two currently popular ones are:

1. *Continuous Slow Running* (*Jogging*) which involves running a long distance at a relatively slow pace is a versatile exercise. You can do it alone or in groups, inside or outside, on a track or down the road, and at any time of day. Not only does it develop the cardiovascular and respiratory systems but exercises the arms as well as the legs, and has a firming effect on muscle groups throughout the body. It is a quick way to get the training effect started. You set the rate at a slow, steady pace, and a distance or length of time that seems appropriate for you.

2. *Rebound-Running.* Jog-bounce (termed rebound-run) on a minitrampoline is a recent (early 1980s) form of aerobic exercise. Manufacturers report that there are beneficial training effects from working on this equipment; also, that the exerciser will have no trauma in the lower extremities. Research in the area is limited, but this type of running is placed in the "moderate exercise" category along with jogging-walking 4-4½ mph and bicycling 8 mph. For the average individual, rebound-running at a rate of about 60 steps per minute should elevate the heart rate to an acceptable work intensity. The duration required will depend upon the intensity.

Walking is a less vigorous method of exercise or training. It is for those who cannot run, choose to not run, or need to work into a conditioning program gradually. The benefits are basically the same as those for running, but it takes longer to achieve a training effect since the heart rate does not rise as high as for more vigorous activities. For those who

Week	Distance (miles)	Goal Time (min.)
1	2	36
2	2	35
3	2	34
4	2	33
5	2	32
6	2	31
7	2	30
8	2	29

are healthy and under 30 years of age the above program for beginners could be use. You should walk at least every other day and, perhaps, perform calisthenics on the "off" days.

At the end of this time you should begin to jog or increase your distance. Remember, to achieve a training effect you must exercise (walk) for 1½ to 2 hours if your heart rate reaches only 110-120 beats per minute.

Dancing can be an effective means of achieving cardiovascular fitness. The concept of moving to music to improve cardiovascular endurance became quite popular in the 1970s. It is called Aerobic dance and involves a series of specially choreographed routines which are combinations of various dance steps and locomotor movements such as running and skipping. If performed regularly and for extended periods of time (45 minutes to an hour), you can achieve a training effect. Jazzercise is another movement routine set to jazz music, which is used to condition the body. The idea of these types of routines is to use music—jazz, rock, pop, or whatever is rhythmic and popular—to set the exercise tempo.

Cooper's Aerobic Program. Dr. Kenneth Cooper, who introduced aerobics to the Americans in the late 1960s, suggests that the unconditioned beginner use a "starter" program. He designed an "Aerobic's Chart Pack" which consists of a variety of activities arranged in categories based on age and fitness level. You are considered to be in good condition if you average 24 (for women) and 30 (for men) points a week; however, if you have a low level of fitness, begin by earning 0-10 points each week and gradually increase the number. Consult Table VIII to determine how long and how far you must work in the selected activities for the first two months of the program. For example, walking (running) a mile 5 times the first week would earn 5 points. If you run a mile 5 different times and rode your bicycle 2 miles during the second week, you would earn a total of 7 points. Remember the cautions: warm-up properly, do not push yourself too fast, and cool-down slowly.

TABLE VIII

Aerobics Chart Pack*
Starter Program
(Under 30 Years of Age)

Week	Activity	Time Goal (min.)	Distance	Freq./ Wk.	Points/ Wk.
1	Running	32:00	2 miles	3	9
	Stair Climbing	10:00	5 round trips (per minute)	5	0
	Bicycling	9:00	2 miles	3	1.5
	Swimming	12:00	300 yards	4	0
2	Running	30:00	2 miles	3	9
	Stair Climbing	10:00	5 round trips (per minute)	5	0
	Bicycling	9:00	2 miles	3	4.5
	Swimming	12:00	300 yards	4	0
3	Running	27:00	2 miles	3	15
	Stair Climbing	10:00	5 round trips (per minute)	5	0
	Bicycling	10:45	3 miles	3	9
	Swimming	10:30	300 yards	4	0
4	Running	26:00	2 miles	3	15
	Stair Climbing	12:00	5 round trips (per minute)	5	0
	Bicycling	10:00	3 miles	4	12
	Swimming	20:00	500 yards	5	0

Notes: Stairs—Applies to 10 steps, 6″ to 7″ in height, 25° to 30° incline. Use of banister is encouraged.
    Swimming—Applies to overhand crawl.
*From *The Aerobics Way* by Kenneth H. Cooper, M.D., M.P.H. Copyright © 1977 by Kenneth Cooper. Reprinted by permission of the publishers, M. Evans & Co., Inc., New York, New York 10017.

Anaerobic Exercises

Anaerobic means "without oxygen." Exercises in this category, as in the aerobic one, place a demand on the cardiovascular and respiratory systems. To improve cardiovascular fitness using anaerobic exercises you must perform above 60 percent of maximum speed for long intervals, or above 90 percent for short intervals, and then walk or jog until the heart rate returns to 120 BPM, continuing for a minimum of 15 to 30 minutes.

TABLE VIII—*Continued*

Week	Activity	Time Goal (min.)	Distance	Freq./ Wk.	Points/ Wk.
5	Running	25:00	2 miles	3	15
	Stair Climbing	12:00	5 round trips (per minute)	5	0
	Bicycling	15:00	4 miles	4	18
	Swimming	18:00	500 yards	5	0
6	Running	24:30	2 miles	3	15
	Stair Climbing	12:00	5 round trips (per minute)	5	0
	Bicycling	14:30	4 miles	4	18
	Swimming	17:00	500 yards	5	0
7	Running	24:00	2 miles	3	21
	Stair Climbing	8:30	6 round trips (per minute)	4	8
	Bicycling	18:30	5 miles	4	24
	Swimming	44:00	200 yards	5	8.35
8	Running	22:00	2 miles	3	21
	Stair Climbing	9:30	6 round trips (per minute)	4	9
	Bicycling	18:00	5 miles	4	24
	Swimming	6:00	300 yards	5	12:5

Interval Running. Involves alternating a work period with a rest period. Three variables are involved: the distance to be run, the time needed to run the distance, and the rest period (either a specified time or distance) between each run. You may alter any of these to arrange your workout so that it consists of alternating sprinting with jogging or walking. You may choose to run 5 repetitions of fifty yards at full speed with a 25 yard jog between each repetition, or run 4 repetitions of 100 yards at full speed with a 20-second walk interval between each of the repetitions. Longer distances can be covered. You may decide to run 2 repetitions of one mile each in 8 minutes, with a 3 minute walk rest interval between the repetitions.

Acceleration Running. Involves moving from jogging to striding, to sprinting, to walking. The distance may vary as you move from the slow pace (jog 30 yards), to a faster pace (stride 30 yards), to moving at full speed for 30 yards. Follow this with 40 or 50 yards of walking before beginning the routine again. Repeat several times.

Strength and Muscular Endurance

Progressive Resistance Exercises

Progressive Resistance Exercises (*P.R.E.*) allow you to develop muscular strength or endurance by precisely and progressively regulating the degree of muscular stress for the specific muscle desired. Both men and women can enjoy and benefit from resistance-producing equipment (such as dumbbells, weight machines, barbells, wall pulleys, and ergometers) for strength and muscular endurance. There has been a misconception that resistance-type exercises would develop unwanted bulging muscles in females. Women's muscles will develop, but since females possess about one-third less muscle mass than their male counterparts, they will not develop a so-called masculine physique. Of course, not all men will be able to develop the "Mr. America" physique, either.

The general principles of progressive resistance exercises are:

1. Low repetitions and high-resistance produce strength.
2. High repetitions and low-resistance produce endurance.
3. Neither of these types of exercises is capable of producing the results obtained by the other type.

Endurance can be gained by performing a high number of repetitions (for example 20 or more repetitions) with light to moderate weights. Select a weight by the trial and error method starting with one-fourth your body weight or the maximum amount of weight that you can lift 20 times through the range of motion in each of three sets. (A *set* means any number of successive repetitions without an intervening rest.) Rest for approximately one-and-one-half to three minutes between sets. When you feel that this is not a sufficient work load, increase the weight. Each muscle group has a different strength capacity, therefore it will be necessary to find the appropriate load for each exercise.

Strength can be significantly increased only by working against a degree of resistance that is near maximal effort. The work load should be lifted for four to ten repetitions. For example, using eight repetitions, find the maximum amount of weight that you can move eight times through the full range of movement. This is called 8-RM (*RM* means "repetition maximum," or the maximum weight which can be raised a specified number of times—eight, in this case—using maximum muscular exertion.) You should strive to complete three sets, staying within the four to ten repetition range. When you are able to exceed 10 repetitions in any of the three sets, the weight should be increased in order once again to exert maximum effort within the four to ten range. A person might do 10 repetitions the first set, six the second set, and only four the last set; but this is adequate for strength training.

Another method is to take one-half of your 8-RM for eight repetitions (½ 8-RM), three-fourths 8-RM the second set, and the full 8-RM for the final set. If the weight were 12 pounds, you would lift six pounds the first set, nine pounds the second set, and 12 pounds the last set. Some prefer this method done in reverse order; i.e., start with 8-RM, then ¾ 8-RM, and finally ½ 8-RM on the third set.

Weight Training Exercises

The best way to use weights is through an individually designed program; do not attempt to duplicate one that has been set-up for someone else. Before attempting to do any exercise with the weights, warm-up slowly and completely. Warm-up the whole body; place special emphasis on the shoulder, back, and knee joints. Be especially careful not to overstrain the back and abdominal muscles. The chance of doing damage in these areas probably is greater than in other areas of the body.

It is vitally important that each exercise be performed throughout the specific muscle group's full range of muscular activity and that each repetition be executed correctly. Each repetition should start from the *prestretched position* (with the muscle elongated) and be executed concentrically (shorten the muscles) for about two seconds and then eccentrically (lengthen the muscles) for about four seconds. Large muscle groups (back, chest, hips, legs) are generally exercised before the smaller muscle groups (neck, elbow, wrist, ankle). There should be a lapse of 48 hours between work bouts.

Do not forget safety. Use spotters, especially on bench presses. Use the "4" rather than the "7" position when lifting—this means flex your knees and hips but keep your back straight ("4") rather than keeping legs straight and bending the back ("7"). Maintain good body alignment: keep your pelvis stabilized. All movements must be executed smoothly; there should be no jerking or heaving. It is customary to exhale during the exertion of the movement and to inhale as the weight is lowered. Do not hold your breath.

Exercises with Barbells. You can find specific exercises for strength or muscular endurance in weight training books and charts that usually accompany a weight machine. These are only a few of the many used to develop these two components of fitness, depending on the resistance and repetitions. (Dumbbells, pulleys, or other resistance can be substituted for many of these.)

Two-arm (Biceps) Curl—used to develop the flexors of the elbow.

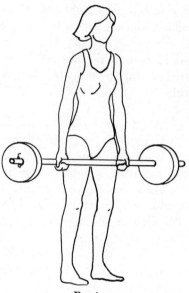

Stand erect, arms at sides
Place feet shoulder width apart
Point toes straight ahead
Face palms forward
Place hands shoulder width apart

Begin

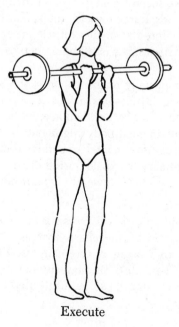

Curl bar slowly and steadily to
    shoulder
Exhale while raising weight
Keep elbows close to but not touch-
    ing body
Return slowly and steadily to start-
    ing position
Inhale while lowering weight

Execute

Upright Rowing—used to develop the flexors of the elbow and the muscles of the shoulders and upper back.

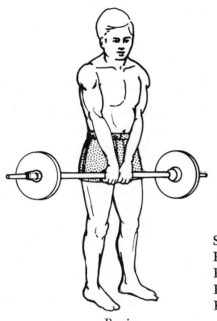

Stand erect
Place feet shoulder width apart
Point toes straight ahead
Face palms toward body
Keep hands close together

Begin

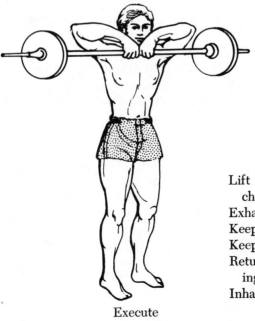

Lift bar slowly and steadily to chin
Exhale while raising weight
Keep bar close to body
Keep elbows higher than hands
Return slowly and steadily to starting position
Inhale while lowering weight

Execute

Bench Press—used to develop extensors of the elbows and flexors of the shoulders and the chest.

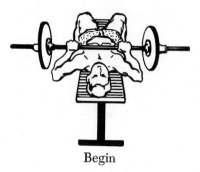

Begin

Have a spotter
Lie supine on a bench
Place feet on floor shoulder width
   apart
Face palms away from body
Place hands about shoulder width
   apart; place thumbs under bar

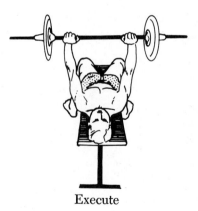

Execute

Push the bar slowly and steadily
   until arms are extended
Exhale on the extension
Return slowly and steadily to start-
   ing position
Inhale while lowering weight

Shoulder Press—is used to develop the arm extensors.

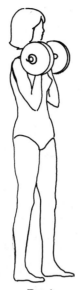

Stand erect
Place feet shoulder width apart
Point toes straight ahead
Face palms away from body
Place hands shoulder width apart

Begin

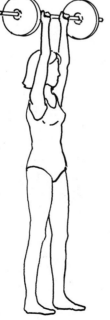

Push the bar slowly and steadily
    until arms are fully extended
Exhale while raising weight
Keep weight in line with center of
gravity
Do not arch back
Return slowly and steadily to start-
    ing position
Inhale while lowering weight

Execute

Half Knee Squats—used to develop the muscles of the upper parts of the thighs.

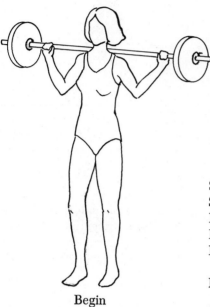

Begin

Stand erect
Spread feet shoulder width apart
Point toes straight ahead
Face palms forward
Place hands farther than shoulder
    width apart
Rest bar on shoulders

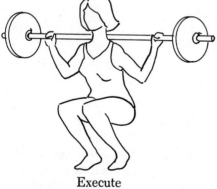

Execute

Squat slowly and steadily
Bend knees to 90° angle
Inhale while body is being lowered
Pause briefly; take several deep
    breaths
Return slowly and steadily to start-
    ing position
Exhale while raising body

Heel-Raises—used to develop the calf muscles in the lower leg.

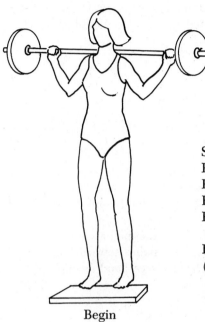

Begin

Stand erect
Place feet shoulder width apart
Point toes in slightly
Face palms forward
Place hands farther apart than
    shoulder width apart
Rest bar on shoulders
(Place balls of feet on two inch
    high board for greater range of
    motion.)

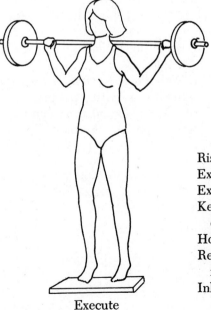

Execute

Rise on tiptoes slowly and steadily
Exhale while raising weight
Extend legs fully
Keep weight over base of support;
    do not lean
Hold for one second
Return slowly and steadily to start-
    ing position
Inhale as weight is lowered

Exercises with Dumbbells. Most exercises that can be performed with a barbell can be duplicated with a dumbbell. The following are two examples. (Tins of food—such as 20 ounces of peaches, sand filled plastic bottles, or books may be substituted for regular dumbbells.)

Side Bends—used to develop lateral flexors.

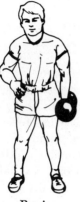

Begin

Stand erect; comfortable side
   stride position
Hold dumbell at side
Face palms toward body
Place free hand on hip

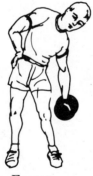

Execute

Bend slowly and steadily to the
   side
Do not lean forward or backward
Return to starting position
Repeat using other arm and bend
   in opposite direction

Flying Motions—used to develop shoulders, upper chest, and back.

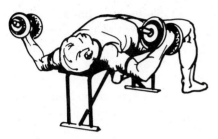

Begin

Lie supine on flat bench
Place feet on floor shoulder width
    apart
Hold dumbells with palms facing
    up
Extend arms in line with shoulders
Partially flex the elbows

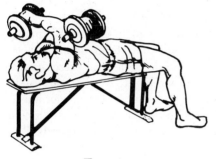

Execute

Cross arms slowly and steadily
    over the chest
Alternate arms in crossing so that
    one is uppermost one time and
    the other the next
Exhale while lifting weight
Return to starting position
Inhale while lowering weight
(Some individuals prefer to alter-
    nate exercises—one arm goes up
    as the other comes down.)

Calisthenics

Calisthenics move the body parts against gravity; they are primarily suitable to develop muscular endurance and flexibility. Some mild strengthing may occur in weaker individuals, but for the most part gravity does not provide sufficient overload for strength development.

These exercises probably number in the thousands, but only a few have been selected for inclusion in this book. Your instructor probably will suggest additional ones, and you may wish to seek still others to vary your program. From those selected to meet your personal needs, you may find that combining them into a fixed daily routine has several advantages. With intelligent selection, the fixed routine allows the important body parts to be exercised regularly. Such a routine saves time by eliminating the "what-shall-I-do today?" decision. Examples of such a routine are the *Adult Physical Fitness Program for Men and Women*[2], the *Royal Canadian Air Force Exercise Plans for Physical Fitness*,[3] and the *P.E.P. Routine* of these routines are interestingly and scientifically conceived. The latter two are included here.

XBX Exercise Plan

The Royal Canadian Air Force (RCAF) designed an exercise plan for women, called the "XBX". It is just as suitable for men, but men will be able to progress faster. The plan consists of four charts of 10 exercises each arranged in progressive order of difficulty. Each chart is divided into 12 performance levels, numbered consecutively from one (the easiest) to 48 (the most difficult). A total of 12 minutes is allowed in which to perform the entire routine, and there is a time limit for each exercise. The number of repetitions of each exercise increases as you advance to higher levels, and the exercises are modified to become more difficult as you move to the next higher chart. Do not skip levels as you progress. A healthy young adult should spend at least one day at each level on Chart I, two days at each level on Chart II, three days at each level on Chart III, etc. Move to a new level when you can perform the routine without undue strain or soreness. When you have reached your maximum level of performance, three exercise periods per week should be adequate to maintain it.

As with all exercise workouts, you should do cool-down exercises after completing the XBX routine. Walking and stretching exercises are useful for this purpose. The exercises are designed to use most of the major muscle groups of the body, and to develop the health related physical fitness components. The primary purposes of each of the exercises are described below.

Purpose of XBX Exercise

1. *Toe Touch*—Flexibility; stretches muscles in lower back and in back of legs.
2. *Knee Raise*—Flexibility; stretches lower back and hip muscles, and helps improve endurance and strength of muscles on the front of the thighs (good for lordosis).
3. *Lateral Bend*—Flexibility and endurance and strength of trunk muscles (waist slimmer).
4. *Arm Circle*—Flexibility; stretches pectoral muscle across chest; also increases endurance and strength of muscles in the upper back. (Good for round shoulders, kyphosis, and sunken chest.)
5. *Sit-ups*—Strengthens abdominals.
6. a. *Chest and Leg Raise*—Increases endurance and strength of back and hip muscles. (Good for kyphosis and slim hips.)
   b. *Knee-to-Nose Touch*—Stretches lower back; improves endurance and strength of upper back and hip muscles.

7. a. *Side Leg Raise*—Increases endurance and strength of muscles on side of hip and thigh (thigh slimmer).
   b. *Leg Over*—Strengthens trunk muscles as well as thigh muscles.
8. *Push-ups*—Increases endurance and strength of chest muscles and back of upper arms.
9. *Leg Lift*—Increases endurance and strength of muscles on front of thigh (thigh slimmer).
10. *Run and Hop, Jump, Knee Bend, or Squat*—Cardiovascular endurance; increases strength and endurance of muscles in legs and hips.

CHART I

LEVEL		EXERCISE									
		1	2	3	4	5	6	7	8	9	10
	12	9	8	10	40	26	20	28	14	14	170
	11	9	8	10	40	24	18	26	13	14	160
	10	9	8	10	40	22	16	25	12	12	150
	9	7	7	8	36	20	14	23	10	11	140
L	8	7	7	8	36	18	12	20	9	10	125
E	7	7	7	8	36	16	12	18	8	10	115
V	6	5	5	7	28	14	10	16	7	8	100
E	5	5	5	7	28	12	8	13	6	6	90
L	4	5	5	7	28	10	8	10	5	6	80
	3	3	4	5	24	8	6	8	4	4	70
	2	3	4	5	24	6	4	6	3	3	60
	1	3	4	5	24	4	4	4	3	2	50
Minutes for each Exercise		2				2	1	1	2	1	3

CHART I

CHART I EXERCISES

1.a. **Toe Touch.** Feet 12″ apart; arms overhead; try to touch floor.
  b. **Alternate.**° Same as above, except perform in sitting position.
2. **Knee Raise.** Raise alternate knees and pull toward chest with arms; keep back straight; left plus right is 1 count.
3. **Lateral Bend.** Feet 12″ apart; alternate sideward, bending to right and left, sliding hand down leg as far as possible; left plus right is 1 count.
4. **Arm Circle.**° Feet 12″ apart; make large backward circles with one arm; half repetitions with left arm, half with right.
5. **Partial Sit-ups.** Back lying; arms at side; raise head and shoulders until you can see your heels.
6.a. **Chest and Leg Raise.** Front lying; hands under thighs; raise head and shoulders and alternate legs as high as possible; left is one count, right is one count.
  b. **Knee-to-Nose Touch.**° (For those with lordosis.) On hands and knees, try to touch nose with knee; then extend leg backward *parallel* with floor while raising head; do not arch back; half of repetitions with right leg, half with left.
7. **Side Leg Raise.** Side lying; use arms for balance; raise upper leg 18-24 inches; half of repetitions left leg, half right.
8. **Push-ups.** Front lying; hands under shoulders; push up and rock back on heels; keep hands and knees on floor; return to starting position.
9. **Leg Lift.** Back lying; arms at side; raise alternate legs perpendicular to floor; left plus right is 1 count.
10. **Run and Hop.** Run in place; lift knees and feet at least 4″ high; left plus right is 1 count; after 50 counts, jump up and down 10 times, lifting feet at least 4″ high.

° Starred exercises are those revised by the authors.
  Those persons with lordosis should perform exercise 6.b. rather than 6.a.

CHART II

		EXERCISE									
		1	2	3	4	5	6	7	8	9	10
	24	15	16	12	30	35	38	50	28	20	210
	23	15	16	12	30	33	36	48	26	18	200
	22	15	16	12	30	31	34	48	24	18	200
	21	13	14	11	26	29	32	44	23	16	190
L	20	13	14	11	26	27	31	42	21	16	175
E	19	13	14	11	26	24	29	40	20	14	160
V	18	12	12	9	20	22	27	38	18	14	150
E	17	12	12	9	20	19	24	36	16	12	150
L	16	12	12	9	20	16	21	34	14	10	140
	15	10	10	7	18	14	18	32	14	10	130
	14	10	10	7	18	11	15	30	10	8	120
	13	10	10	7	18	9	12	28	8	8	120
Minutes for each Exercise				2		2	1	1	2	1	3

CHART II

CHART II EXERCISES—(Same as Chart I, except as noted.)
1. **Toe Touch.** Bob once, touching floor a second time.
2. **Knee Raise.**
3. **Lateral Bend.** Bob once, sliding hand down leg a second time.
4. **Arm Circle.*** Circle both arms backward simultaneously.
5. **Rocking Sit-ups.** Back lying with knees bent; arms overhead; swing arms and sit up while legs extend; try to touch toes; return to starting position.
6.a. **Chest and Leg Raise.** Lift head and shoulders and both legs at same time.
  b. **Knee-to-Nose Touch.***
7. **Side Leg Raise.** Try to raise leg perpendicular to floor.
8. **Knee Push-ups.** Keep body line straight while pushing up and down; do not rock back on heels.
9. **Leg Overs.** Back lying; arms out at shoulder level; raise one leg to perpendicular and try to touch opposite hand with toes; return to perpendicular and to starting position; alternate legs; left is 1 count; right is 1 count.
10. **Run-and-Stride Jump.** Do 10 jumping-jacks after every 50 runs.

* Starred exercises are those revised by the authors.
  Those persons with lordosis should perform exercise 6.b. rather than 6.a.

CHART III

		EXERCISE									
		1	2	3	4	5	6	7	8	9	10
	36	15	22	18	40	42	40	60	40	20	240
	35	15	22	18	40	41	39	60	39	20	230
	34	15	22	18	40	40	38	58	37	19	220
	33	13	20	16	36	39	36	58	35	19	210
L	32	13	20	16	36	37	36	56	34	18	200
E	31	13	20	16	36	35	34	56	32	16	200
V	30	12	18	14	30	33	33	54	30	15	190
E	29	12	18	14	30	32	31	54	29	14	180
L	28	12	18	14	30	31	30	52	27	12	170
	27	10	16	12	24	29	30	52	25	11	160
	26	10	16	12	24	27	29	50	23	9	150
	25	10	16	12	24	26	28	48	22	8	140
Minutes for each Exercise		2				2	1	1	2	1	3

CHART III

CHART III EXERCISES—(Same as Chart II, except as noted.)
1. **Toe Touch.** Feet 16″ apart; arms overhead; bob, and touch floor to left, center,and right.
2. **Knee Raise.**
3. **Lateral Bend.** Raise one arm overhead with elbow bent; bend and reach to opposite side; alternate sides.
4. **Arm Circle.°** Alternate arms backward like a windmill; left plus right is 1 count.
5. **Sit-ups.°** Back lying with knees bent, arms at sides, feet not held.
6.a. **Chest and Leg Raise.** Arms stretched sideward at shoulder level; lift arms, head, shoulders, and both legs simultaneously.
   b. **Knee-to-Nose Touch.°**
7. **Side Leg Raise.°**
8. **Elbow Push-ups.°** ....Front lying; elbows under shoulders; forearms on floor with hands clasped; raise hips from floor until body line is straight and supported by forearms and toes; rock forward and backward from toes, bringing upper arms near forearms; keep back straight.
9. **Legs-Over Tuck.** Back lying; bend knees to chest; keep shoulders on floor and roll, touching tucked knees to floor on left, then right for 1 count; keep knees together and near chest throughout; return to starting position.
10. **Run and Half-Knee Bends.** After 50 runs raising feet 6″ high, do 10 half-knee bends with hands on hips; 90-110° angle of knee flexion.

° Starred exercises are those revised by the authors.
Those persons with lordosis should perform exercise 6.b. rather than 6.a.

CHART IV

		EXERCISE									
		1	2	3	4	5	6	7	8	9	10
	48	15	26	15	32	48	46	58	30	16	230
	47	15	26	15	32	45	45	56	27	15	220
	46	15	26	15	32	44	44	54	24	14	210
	45	13	24	14	30	42	43	52	21	13	200
L	44	13	24	14	30	40	42	50	19	13	190
E	43	13	24	14	30	38	40	48	16	12	175
V	42	12	22	12	28	35	39	46	13	10	160
E	41	12	22	12	28	32	38	44	11	9	150
L	40	12	22	12	28	30	38	40	9	8	140
	39	10	20	10	26	29	36	38	8	7	130
	38	10	20	10	26	27	35	36	7	6	115
	37	10	20	10	26	25	34	34	6	5	100
Minutes for each Exercise			2			2	1	1	2	1	3

CHART IV

CHART IV EXERCISES—(Same as Chart III, except as noted.)
1. **Toe Touch.** Bob left, center, right.
2. **Knee Raise.**
3. **Lateral Bend.** Arm overhead; bob a second time to each side.
4. **Arm Fling.** Feet 12″ apart; elbows up and out; finger tips touching in front of chest; jerk elbows back and return to start; fling arms back as far as possible, straightening elbow; keep the jerk and fling high; each fling counts 1.
5. **Sit-ups.** Back lying with knees bent, arms crossed on chest; feet not held.
6.a. **Chest and Leg Raise.** Hands clasped behind neck.
   b. **Knee-to-Nose Touch.**°
7. **Side Leg Raise.** Right side toward floor; weight supported on right hand (arm straight) and side of right foot; left arm for balance; *keep body line straight* and raise left leg parallel to floor; half of repetitions on right side, half on left.
8. **Push-ups.** Body line straight from shoulders to toes; do push-ups from toes touching chest each time.
9. **Legs-Over Straight.**° Bend both knees to chest, then raise legs perpendicular to floor; keep shoulders on floor and roll, trying to touch feet to hand on each side; return to perpendicular, then starting position; left plus right is 1 count.
10. **Run and Semi-Squat Jump.** After each 50 runs, do 10 semi-squat jumps by half crouching, with hands on knees, arms straight; one foot slightly ahead of other; jump so feet leave floor and body is erect; land with feet in reverse position.

° Starred exercises are those revised by the authors.
   Those persons with lordosis should perform exercise 6.b. rather than 6.a.

Progressive Exercise Plan for Men (P.E.P.). These exercises are designed for men but could be utilized by women. The routine consists of 10 exercises arranged in progressive order of difficulty. As with the XBX Plan, each chart is divided into 12 performance levels numbered from one (the easiest) to 12 (the most difficult). There is a time limit for each exercise; the complete routine is to be completed in 11 minutes—10 minutes of exercising and a minute of changing between exercises. It may be necessary to find a beginning point by trial and error method. If you are a reasonably active, healthy, young man you would begin at a higher level than one who is older or inactive. Begin at a level at which you can perform the exercises correctly and without undue strain and soreness. It may be necessary to spend several days at each level; spend at least one day. Move to a higher level only when you are completing the present exercises within the established time frame, without becoming too breathless. After reaching your desired level of performance, three workout periods a week should be sufficient to maintain it.

Purpose of P.E.P. Exercises. The plan is designed to use most of the major muscle groups of the body and to develop the health related physical fitness components. The primary purposes of each exercise are:

1. Toe Touch and Knee Touch—(See XBX 1)
2. Knee Raise—(See XBX 2)
3. Trunk Twist—(See XBX 3)
4. Arm Circle—(See XBX 4)
5. Sit-ups—(See (XBX 5)
6. a. Knee-to-Nose Touch—(See XBX6b)
   b. Hip Raise—Stretches muscles in the lower back and in back of legs; improves endurance and strength of arms and shoulders.
7. Modified Splits—Increases endurance and strength of abductors and adductors of thigh, increases flexibility of adductors.
8. Push-ups—(See XBX 8).
9. Flutter Kick—Increases strength and endurance of the hip extensor muscles (especially gluteals and hamstrings).
10. Run and Jump—(See XBX 10).

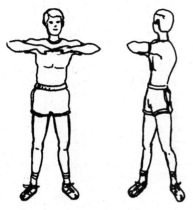

P.E.P. Chart I: Trunk Twist

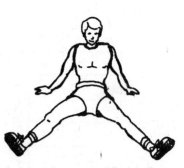

P.E.P. Chart I: Modified Splits

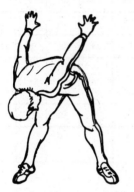

P.E.P. Chart II: Knee Touch

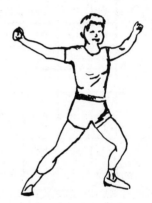

Continuous Exercise: Step and Reach
(Table IX No. 2)

P.E.P.

CHART I

		EXERCISE									
		1	2	3	4	5	6	7	8	9	10
	12	25	30	25	35	50	30	50	50	40	280
	11	24	29	24	34	48	29	48	48	38	275
	10	23	28	23	33	46	28	46	46	36	270
	9	22	27	22	32	44	27	44	44	34	265
L	8	21	26	21	31	42	26	42	42	32	260
E	7	20	25	20	30	40	25	40	40	30	255
V	6	19	24	19	29	38	24	38	38	28	250
E	5	18	23	18	28	36	23	36	36	26	240
L	4	17	22	17	27	34	22	34	34	24	230
	3	16	21	16	26	32	21	32	32	22	220
	2	15	20	15	25	30	20	30	30	20	210
	1	14	19	14	24	28	19	28	28	18	200
Time (min.)		½	½	½	½	1	1	1	1	1	3

CHART I EXERCISES

1. Toe Touch. Stand with feet 12″ apart; arms overhead; try to touch floor, bob once, touching floor a second time.
2. Knee Raise. Stand with feet 6″ apart; raise alternate knees and pull toward chest with arms; keep back straight; left plus right is 1 count.
3. Trunk Twist. Stand with feet shoulder width apart; place hands in front of chest; keep elbows shoulder height; right, left, right, etc. left plus right is 1 count.
4. Arm Circle. Stand with feet 12″ apart, circle both arms backward simultaneously.
5. Sit-ups. Back lying with knees bent; arms overhead; swing arms overhead and sit up while legs extend; touch toes and return to starting position.
6. Knee-to-nose Touch. On hands and knees, try to touch nose with knee; extend leg parallel with floor while raising head; do not arch back; half of repetitions with right leg, half with left.
7. Modified Splits. Sit with legs extended in front; feet together; place hands 6″ behind buttocks and lean back; move left leg to the side and back to starting position; repeat with right leg; left plus right is 1 count.
8. Push-ups. Rest weight on hands and knees; keep body in line while pushing up and down; do not rock back on heels; up and down is 1 count.
9. Flutter Kick. Front lying; hands tucked under thighs; flutter kick, kick from the hips with knees slightly bent; move the legs about 8″ vertically. Each kick is 1 count.
10. Run and Jump. Run in place; lift feet approximately 4″ off the floor; left plus right is 1 count; after 75 counts do 10 jumping jacks; repeat sequence.

P.E.P.
CHART II

		EXERCISE									
		1	2	3	4	5	6	7	8	9	10
	24	25	30	25	40	60	38	50	50	50	260
	23	24	28	24	39	58	36	48	48	48	250
	22	23	28	23	38	56	34	46	46	46	240
	21	22	26	22	37	54	32	44	44	44	230
L	20	21	26	21	36	52	30	42	42	42	220
E	19	20	24	20	35	50	28	40	40	40	210
V	18	18	24	19	34	48	26	38	38	38	200
E	17	18	23	18	33	46	24	36	36	36	190
L	16	17	23	17	32	44	22	34	34	34	180
	15	16	22	16	31	42	20	32	32	32	170
	14	15	21	15	30	40	18	30	30	30	160
	13	14	20	14	29	38	16	28	28	28	150
Time (min.)		½	½	½	½	1	1	1	1	1	3

CHART II EXERCISES
1. Knee Touch. Feet 12″ apart; arms at sides; fling arms behind while bending down from waist with head towards left knee; bob once; return to starting position; repeat with right knee; left plus right is 1 count.
2. Knee Raise.
3. Trunk Twist.
4. Arm Circle. Alternate arms backward like a windmill; left plus right is 1 count.
5. Sit-ups. Back lying with knees bent; arms crossed and hands placed on shoulders; feet not held.
6. Hip Raise. Hands and feet on ground; legs straight; hips in the air; head between arms; bring hips down and head up with a rocking movement; return to starting position. Up and down is 1 count.
7. Modified Splits. Sit with legs extended (feet together) forward; place hands 6″ behind buttocks and lean back; split legs outward; return to starting position.
8. Push-ups. Front lying; palms flat on floor; body line straight from shoulders to toes; straighten arms; touch chest to floor for each completed count.
9. Flutter Kick.
10. Run and Jump. Lift knees waist high. After each 75 counts do 10 semi-spread-eagle jumps by half crouching with hands on knees, arms straight; jump up, raise arms to side and shoulder level, spread feet at least shoulder width apart; land with feet together and arms at sides; repeat sequence.

TABLE IX
Continuous Exercise Routine
(could be set to music)

Exercise	Time (min.)	Activity	Description
1	½	Body Bender	See page 59
2	1	Step and Reach	Stand with arms at sides. Take a long step forward with right foot and reach forward with arms; repeat with left foot. Step to the side with the right foot and raise the arms sideward; repeat with left foot. Step backwards with the right foot and reach the arms backwards; repeat with left foot. Repeat as time permits.
3	½	Overhead Reach/ Toe Touch	Stand on tiptoes and reach high 5 times; touch fingers to toes or floor 5 times. (Repeat if time permits.)
4	2	Walk/Jog	Walk 2 gym laps; jog 2 laps. Breathe deeply; swing arms briskly. (Repeat if time permits.)
5	1	Push-ups	See pages 4 and 5
6	½	Arm Flings	See page 58
7	½	Jumping Jacks	
8	1	Roll Downs	See page 57
9	3	Walk/Skip/Gallop	Walk 1 lap at a fast pace; skip 1 lap; gallop 1 lap. Repeat if time permits.
10	1	High Stepper	Stand erect with elbows bent and hands relaxed. Walk in place; lift feet about a foot off the floor and pump arms vigorously.
11	½	Ankle Write	See page 114
12	½	Knee-to-Nose Kick	See XBX Chart I, 6b
13	3	Jog	Jog at medium pace.
14	2	Walk	Walk at medium pace. Breathe deeply; swing arms briskly.
15	1	Calf Stretcher	See page 60
16	1	Knee Raise	See XBX Chart I, II
17	1	Mad Cat	See page 121

Selected Exercises for Physical Fitness

The repetitions noted for each exercise are suggested beginning levels. Start at this level and gradually increase the repetitions.

Strength and Endurance

Arms and Shoulders

1. *Push-ups*—Assume the push-up position. Lower your body until your chest touches the floor, and return to the starting position, keeping your body straight. Repeat five times.
2. *Pull-ups*—Hang (palms forward and shoulder width apart) from a low bar (may be placed across two chairs), heels on floor, with the body suspended at about a 45 degree angle. Pull up, keeping the body rigid, and touch your chest to the bar. Lower to the starting position. Repeat three times.
3. *Isometric hand pull*—Tailor sit or stand. Keeping the arms at shoulder level, place hands under chin, with fingers extended. Turn one hand palm up and lock fingertips. Keeping the fingertips locked, try to pull the elbows apart. Hold for six seconds, relax, and repeat three times per day.

Abdominals

1. *Roll-downs*—(For persons who can not do sit-ups) Sit with the knees bent and the feet together. Fold your arms across your chest and roll down slowly, keeping the chin tucked to the chest. Relax on the floor, and then sit up any way you choose. Repeat 10 times. (If you cannot do No. 3, do this one.)
2. *Sit-ups* (see chapter 1). Repeat eight times.
3. *Reverse Sit-ups*—Lie on your back, bend the knees, place the feet flat on the floor with arms at sides. Lift the knees to the chest, raising the hips off the floor. Return to the starting position. You may raise the knees toward the right shoulder and then to the left shoulder. Repeat four times.
4. *Pelvic Tilt*—Assume a supine position, with the knees bent and slightly apart. "Press" the spine down on the floor and hold for six seconds— tighten the abdominals and gluteals. Repeat three times, three times per day.
5. *Abdominal and Gluteal Set* (also for legs)—Stand tall, with the feet together, arms hanging loosely at the sides. Tighten the abdominals, gluteals, and thigh muscles. Keep the knees stiff, and tip the body.

Legs

1. *Stationary Leg Change*—Crouch on the floor, with your weight on your hands, left leg bent under the chest, right leg extended behind you. Alternate legs—bring right leg up while left leg goes back. Repeat, alternating right and left, 16 times.
2. *Stride Squat*—Stand tall, feet together. Take a long step forward with the left foot, touching the right knee to the floor. Return to the starting position, and step out with the other foot. Repeat, alternating left and right, eight times.
3. *Flat-foot Rock*—Stand in a wide side-stride position, with the toes pointing outward and the hands on the hips. Lower into a "squat" (knees flexed 90°) over one foot while keeping the other leg straight. Keep the feet in the same spot, and transfer the body from a "squat" over one foot to a "squat" over the other. Do not raise the body while changing position. Repeat, alternating right and left, four times.
4. *Isometric Leg Extensor*—Stand on a jump rope in a side-stride position with back erect, knees slightly flexed, and hands grasping rope at about knee level. Keep the back erect and arms straight while making at attempt to straighten your knees by pulling directly upward on the rope. Hold for six seconds, relax, and repeat three times, three times per day.
5. *Modified Knee Bends*—Stand in a side-stride position with feet about six inches apart. Kneel on the right knee while maintaining good posture. Return to starting position by extending left leg. Kneel on the right knee 5 times in succession. Repeat with left knee. Do not flex the supporting knee more than 90°. (You can maintain balance by holding on to something if you lack sufficient strength.)

Flexibility
Chest, Shoulders, Upper Back
(See pages 95 and 106)

1. *Arm Fling*—Tailor sit or stand. Bend the elbows, keeping the arms at shoulder level and the palms down, under the chin. Push the elbows back, trying to bring the shoulder blades together, then return to starting position. Extend the arms, keeping them at shoulder level, and swing them behind you. Return to original position. Repeat set four times. Keep your chin tucked and your head back.
2. *Prone Elbow Lift*—Lie in a prone position. Place the hands in the small of the back, palms upward. Raise the elbows and shoulders without moving the trunk and head; hold for four counts. Relax and repeat four times.

3. *Hand Raiser*—Sit on a bench or stool with your back against the wall. Keep the arms extended and raise them sideward to shoulder height. Flex the elbows to ninety degree angles, with palms facing downward toward the floor. Slowly lift the hands to touch the wall with the backs of the hands. Hold for four seconds; then slowly lower the hands to touch the wall with the palms. Hold for four seconds; slowly return the hands to shoulder height. Keep the elbows at shoulder height and at 90° angles throughout the movement. Relax and repeat four times.
4. *Shoulder Stretch*—Tailor sit or stand. Reach the right hand over the left shoulder and the left hand upward behind your back, and try to hook the fingers. Reverse, reaching with the left hand over the left shoulder and the right hand behind your back. Repeat four times.
5. *Inverted*—T—Assume a hook-lying position. Place the hands (palms up) on the floor and the elbows (flexed at a 90° angle) at shoulder height. Keep the backs of the hands and the elbows on the floor while slowly sliding the arms down until the elbows touch your rib cage. Repeat four times.

Waist and Trunk
1. *Lateral Stretch*—Stand in a side-stride position. Raise your right arm overhead, and lean to the left as you reach across your body with your left arm. "Reach" in opposite directions four times. Alternate with the right side.
2. *Torso Twist*—Stand in a side-stride position, with your arms raised to the side at shoulder level. Keep your hips facing forward, as your upper trunk and head "twist" to the left until your right arm is extended forward and your left arm is extended backward. Return to the starting position, and then twist to the right side. Your eyes should follow the hand that is behind you. Repeat four sets.
3. *Body Bender*—Stand in a side-stride position, with the hands behind your neck and the fingers interlaced. Bend the trunk *sideward* to the left as far as possible; return to the starting position; bend the trunk *sideward* to the right. Repeat four sets.
4. *Knee Over*— Lie supine with the legs extended, arms at the sides. Slide the right foot up until the lower leg is perpendicular to the floor. Keeping your shoulders in contact with the floor, try to touch the floor beside your left hip with your right knee. Return to the initial position and repeat with the left knee. Alternating legs, repeat six sets.

Lower Back and Legs
(See pages 106-107)

1. *Hamstring Stretch*—Sit on floor with legs extended. Bend your right knee and rest the sole of the right foot against the inside left thigh. Lean forward and grasp the ankle of the left foot with both hands. Hold an easy stretch for 30 to 40 seconds. Relax, then repeat. Repeat actions with other leg.
2. *Back Stretch*—Lie on your right side with the legs extended. Grasp right knee with hands and pull to chest; return to the starting position and repeat four times. Repeat on the left side with left knee.
3. *Knee-to-Nose Kick*—On hands and knees, bring your right knee to your nose, and then kick the leg out backwards as you lift your head. Repeat four times, and then change to the left leg. Repeat four sets. (Students with lordosis should not raise the leg above the level of the hips.)
4. *Sprinter's Crouch*—Squat, place the hands on the floor in line with the shoulders, and point the fingers forward. Extend the left leg fully to the rear. Bounce hips up and down four times; reverse the legs, and repeat with the right leg extended. Repeat four sets.
5. *Ground Hurdling*—Sit with one leg extended forward, and the other flexed at the knee so that the foot is at the side and slightly behind the body. Flex your trunk as much as possible, and reach with both hands for the toes of the extended leg. Repeat six times. Reverse the legs and repeat.
6. *Calf Stretch*—Stand arms length away from a solid support. Place forearms on the support and rest your head on your hands. Place the left foot between you and the support; bend the knee. Keep the toes of both feet pointing to the support and the heels in contact with the floor. Move hips slowly forward until you feel your calf stretch. Hold an easy stretch for 30 to 40 seconds. Relax, repeat action. Repeat actions with other leg.
7. *Leg Raise*—Lie in a supine position with the legs extended. Slowly raise the left leg to 90° angle. Flex the knee and bring it to the chest. Extend the knee, and lower the leg slowly to the floor, Alternating legs, repeat eight sets.

Selected Exercises for Figure/Physique Improvement

Bust/Chest

The breasts are glands, not muscles; therefore, exercises for the bust are of doubtful value. However, exercises which improve the strength of the chest muscles (pectorals) supporting the bust, combined with good posture can help a woman appear well endowed. Strangely enough, the same exercise may help decrease the measurements of those who are over-endowed, but you should be realistic in your expectations; exercises will not make the big person small nor the small, big. Men should use the same exercises to improve their posture and physique.

Push-ups are good exercises for this purpose. Backward arm circling will help improve your upper trunk posture. A more specific exercise is done by holding the arms in front of you and clasping your wrists. Push and pull strongly toward and away from your elbows. Feel the skin on your arms sliding and the chest muscles contracting as you push/pull. The *bench press* develops the pectoral muscles, also.

Waist

The front half of your waist is made up of the abdominal muscles so abdominal strengthening exercises, such as isometrics and sit-ups, are the most effective waist exercises. To develop all of the muscles, however, execute your sit-ups with a twist to the right and left. These same exer-cises will help rid you of abdominal ptosis. An exercise to help strengthen the side and back muscles (at the same time they are increasing flexibility), consists of holding a weight in one hand and bending the trunk sideward in the opposite direction. If your waist is big because of fat, these local exercises will not reduce the fat. Men tend to deposit fat here and develop a "pot."

Hips

To firm flabby hips you need to exercise the buttocks muscles (gluteus maximus) which cross the hip joint at the back. This can be accomplished by simply tightening the seat isometrically. *Prone leg lifts, knee-to-nose kicks, and leg exercises* on page 48 are appropriate. (Also, see back exer-cises in Chapter 7).

For most women it is the padding (sometimes known as "Saddlebags") on the sides of the hips that is of the most concern. Just remember that it is the "nature of the female species" to have a broad pelvis and fat deposits on the hips and thighs. Strengthening the gluteus maximus and minimus and other muscles that cross the side of the hip joint will help tighten the flab in that region. *Side leg raises* (See XBX exercise VII) are useful for this purpose, as are *isometric contractions. Running, rope jump-ing, stair climbing,* and *jumping jacks* also employ the hip muscles.

Calf

Men, more than women sometimes want to develop a larger calf muscle. *Running* and *jumping* help, but, more specifically, exercises which cause toe-pointing against resistance will strengthen the calf muscle. *Tip-toeing* with weights on the shoulders or in the hands is one example.

Thighs

Hip exercises are useful for strengthening (and therefore, firming) the thighs, but to that list you might add *leg circling*. Lie supine and raise one leg to make a 90° angle with the hip (avoid arching the back). Move it in clockwise and counterclockwise circles, or write your name and address in the air. Keep your leg straight; make the movement from the hip joint. This is more effective if ankle weights are used. *Knee extensions* on a weight training machine will develop the quadriceps muscles.

The muscles on the inside of the thigh, the adductors, are particularly prone to flabbiness because they are rarely used vigorously in everyday activity. *Horseback riding* and *swimming the breaststroke* bring them into play, but these sports are not enjoyed by all. Specifically for that region, try an isometric contraction by sitting on the floor and placing your feet on the outside of a chair. *Squeeze*—try to push the chair legs together. Or sit facing a partner in stride position and try to push their legs together. A *side-lying leg lift* using the bottom leg rather than the top is effective, especially with ankle weights added.

Upper Arms

For men who want more bulky muscles, or for women who wish to get rid of flabby arms and increase strength, the *triceps curl* (elbow extension) or *biceps curl* (elbow flexion) against resistance (pulleys, dumbbells, etc.) are the most popular exercises.

References

1. "News You Can Use In Your Personal Planning," *U.S. News & World Report*, May 1, 1978, p. 93.
2. President's Council of Physical Fitness, *Adult Physical Fitness* (Washington: Superintendent of Documents, U.S. Government Printing Office).
3. Royal Canadian Air Force, *Royal Canadian Air Force Exercise Plans for Physical Fitness* (Ottawa, Canada: Queen's Printer). Used by special arrangement with *This Week Magazine* (New York: United Newspapers Magazine Corp).

Facts about Weight, Fatness, and Nutrition

4

America has a greater abundance of food than any other country in the world—it is also more highly mechanized, with labor saving devices which decrease the need for energy expenditure. Is it any wonder that half of our population is overfat, and that eating and dieting are adult preoccupations? Engineers have calculated that if all of that excess fat were converted to an equal quantity of fuel oil, it would supply the electrical needs of Orange County, California for 100 days!

Doctors are not in agreement as to what constitutes over or under weight, but probably 10 percent over and 10-15 percent under the optimum weight should be cause for concern. The optimum weight of an individual may be estimated from height-weight-age tables, such as Table IV; or, better yet, if you can find an expert to measure your skinfold with calipers, you will be able to evaluate the much more meaningful "percentage of body fat," to determine your leanness.

Weight and fatness control begins with good nutrition. You should make an evaluation of the type and amount of food you consume in order to determine whether it is serving your body needs (see sample Charts VII and VIII in the Appendix).

Before you read this chapter, test yourself on your knowledge of nutrition and weight control by taking the quiz on Chart VI, in the Appendix.

Balanced Diet

The essential components in a balanced diet are vitamins, minerals, protein, fats and oils, carbohydrates, water, roughage, and calories. These are found in the four food groups recommended for the daily diet.

1. *Dairy Products* (*milk and cheese*)—two or more servings.
2. *Meat, Fish, and Eggs* (*protein group*)—two or more servings.
3. *Vegetables and Fruits*—four or more servings.
4. *Breads and Cereals* (*grain products*)—four or more servings.

It has been estimated that six out of ten youth between the ages of 13 and 19 are malnourished. This does not mean that they are underfed, but rather that they are not eating balanced diets. Teenagers have an affinity for pop, candy, and corn chips; but this puts their health in jeopardy, their complexion in a mess and their bodies in the shape of a pear.

The Food and Nutrition Board of the National Academy of Sciences recommends a daily dietary allowance for normal persons living in the United States under normal environmental stresses. As an example, for a woman weighing 128 pounds, height 64", age 18-35, it recommends 2,000 calories; protein 55 grams; calcium 0.8 grams; iron 8 milligrams;vitamin A 5,000 international units; thiamin 1.0 milligrams; riboflavin 1.5 milligrams; niacin 13 milligrams, and ascorbic acid 55 milligrams. For a man weighing 154 pounds, height 69", age 18-35, it recommends 2800 calories; protein 65 grams; calcium 8 grams; iron 10 milligrams; vitamin A, 5000 international units; thiamin 1.4 milligrams; riboflavin 1.7 milligrams; niacin 18 milligrams and ascorbic acid 60 milligrams.

The recommended daily dietary allowance will, in most cases, exceed the minimum daily requirement and if the nutrients mentioned here are taken care of, the 40 or so other less important ones will be, also.

Proteins build and repair the body and provide energy. Ten to 15 percent of the daily caloric requirement should be provided by protein; good sources include eggs, fish, meat, poultry and dairy products.

Carbohydrates furnish energy. The exact amount of carbohydrates needed in the daily diet is not known, however the National Research Council suggests that normal adults require about 500 carbohydrate calories daily; most people far exceed this amount. Carbohydrate food should be selected for its vitamin and mineral content as well as for its caloric content. Such foods include fruits, starchy vegetables, and whole grain cereals.

Fats furnish energy. Many nutritionists recommend that 25-30 percent of one's caloric intake should be composed of fats. The normal diet probably provides at least the minimum amount of fat from meat and vegetable sources.

Minerals such as calcium and iron build and repair the body and regulate its processes. Good sources of calcium include fish, cheese, eggs, poultry, milk, yogurt, fresh fruits, and whole grains. Generous amounts of iron may be found in liver, green vegetables, egg yolk, turkey, beef, oysters, and clams.

Vitamins A, B-complex (thiamin, riboflavin, and niacin), C, and D also regulate the body's processes. Good sources of Vitamin A include liver, cheese, corn, egg yolk, broccoli, sunflower seeds, tomatoes, and peas. The vitamin B-complexes are most abundant in liver, kidneys, cheese, egg yolk, fish, poultry, yogurt, and whole grains. Foods generous in Vitamin C include citrus fruits, cantelope, corn, green vegetables, tomatoes, peas, and potatoes. The sunshine vitamin-D, is prominent in milk, eggs, liver, fish, and oysters.

Causes of Weight and Fatness Problems

Obesity means a body composition of 20 percent or more fat. The *over-fat* person is usually (but not always) also *overweight*. Obesity is a complex medical problem with multiple causes. Some people over-eat for psychological reasons; others have poor eating habits because of family or cultural influences. There are those individuals who simply are ignorant about calories, and in rare instances a person may over-eat because of diminished taste-bud discrimination. Only about 5 percent of the overweight population suffers from metabolic disturbances which predispose them to accumulating fat.

Underweight is probably equally complex. Often it is accompanied by high metabolic levels; nervousness, hyperactivity, or poor eating habits may play a role; abnormal food absorption or loss of calories through urine (as in diabetes) occur in rare cases; sometimes it is an inherited somatotype.

Regardless of the underlying causes, the jokers are right when they say overweight is caused by two things, "chewing and swallowing." Overweight and overfat is the result of consuming more calories than are burned; underweight is the result of consuming fewer calories than are burned ("not swallowing?"). Maintaining proper weight is a matter of balancing input (calories) with output (activity). If the number of calories eaten equals the number burned, weight remains the same. When input exceeds output, weight is gained and deposited in the form of adipose tissue (fat). The distribution of this extra padding is controlled genetically and hormonally. Usually such tissue accumulates around the hips and thighs on women. Men tend to deposit it around the waist.

Why Maintain Proper Weight

All of us are interested in appearance. We want to have a good figure/physique to look good in our clothes, and to be able to wear the latest fashions. While proper weight does not insure good body proportions and good posture, it helps—and an attractive appearance helps increase self-confidence and poise. More important than the psychological rewards are the physiological (health) benefits. Being lean means we are less susceptible to certain diseases and have a better chance to live longer.

Dangers of Obesity

Obesity increases one's susceptibility to a long list of health hazards: respiratory difficulties; cardiac enlargement; congestive heart failure; high blood pressure; hirsutism; difficulties during anesthesia, surgery, pregnancy, and childbirth, varicose veins; osteoarthritis; and gall bladder disease, to name a few. Recently it has been discovered that there is a greater risk of breast cancer in obese women and a poorer chance of recovery. In addition, social pressures may result in the development of neurosis, with an obsessive concern with body image, passivity, withdrawal, and expectation of rejection. The mortality rate for markedly overweight men is 79 percent greater than for those of average weight. For markedly overweight women, it is 61 percent greater. Moderate overweight increases the death rate for men and women to 42 percent greater than normal.

Dangers of Being too Thin

In the past, it was thought that it was healthy to be skinny and that underweight persons outlived us all. New research studies now suggest that underweight people also have higher death rates than people whose weight is normal. This was especially true of those who were at least 20 percent underweight. The exact cause of this increased mortality is not known at this time.

Determination of Caloric Needs

The number of calories needed to maintain proper weight is a very individual matter and depends upon a number of factors: (1) *size*—height, bone size, and muscle mass; (2) *basal metabolic rate*—the BMR is determined by glandular function, is higher in men than women, and decreases with age; (3) *age*—activity and metabolism decrease with age, so about 5 percent fewer calories are needed each 10 years after age 25 (the average age when growth ceases); (4) *activity*—the number of calories burned depends upon how many muscles are used; whether they are large or small muscles; how fast, how hard, and how long the activity is continued; (5) *climate*—more calories are burned in colder climate; (6) *pregnancy;* (7) *lactation;* and (8) *temperament*—highstrung people burn more calories than relaxed people. The National Foods and Nutrition Board has made charts for estimating caloric needs based on these factors, but a quick method of estimating an individual's needs is based on the fact that the *average person needs about 15 calories per pound of body weight.* You can figure your approximate needs by multiplying 15 times your optimum weight to estimate what is required to maintain that weight. Keep in mind the eight factors mentioned previously, and remember it is only an estimate. The only satisfactory method of determining your need is to ascertain whether you are maintaining your proper weight on that amount—if so, then that is the number of calories you need. If your weight is moving in the wrong direction, either your activity or both your activity and caloric input should be adjusted.

The Role of Exercise in Weight and Fatness Control

One pound of fat is equal to about 3500 calories. To lose a pound in a week, you must cut down or burn 3500 calories per week or 500 calories per day. You would have to walk approximately 35 miles to burn one pound of fat. It would take about five hours of walking to get rid of one piece of pie—a half hour of bicycling to burn up one coke—an hour of steady dancing to burn up one piece of cake! But do not be discouraged; it is not necessary to do it in a day. If you take a daily half-hour walk, you could lose 10 pounds in a year. A half hour of tennis or badminton daily could result in a loss of 16 pounds in a year. *Exercise does burn calories* plus helping to maintain muscle tone and prevent flabbiness as weight is lost. Table X is an energy expenditure chart which may be helpful in determining the number of calories burned in some of your every day activities or sports.

It should be obvious that the heavier the person, the more calories burned. If you use the table to estimate your caloric expenditure, remember that the calculations are based on an hour's activity. If you wish to calculate expenditure per minute, multiply your weight times the number of calories per hour and then divide by 60. If you then exercise for only twenty minutes, multiply the caloric expenditure per minute by 20.

Another and perhaps more important reason for exercising is to avoid loss of muscle tissue during weight loss. Studies show that if you diet and do not exercise, you will lose both fat tissue and lean body mass. This loss of muscle (body protein) can not be prevented by increasing protein in the diet. When one loses weight by exercise alone or by a combination of diet and exercise, the weight loss is fat only and there is an increase in lean body mass.

This is illustrated in a study in which three groups of adult women had a 500 calorie per day deficit, either by cutting calorie intake, increasing activity, or both.[1]

	Lost Body Weight	Lost Body Fat	Lost or Gained Lean Body Tissue
Diet Group	−11.7	− 9.3	−2.4
Exercise Group	−10.6	−12.6	+2.0
Exercise-Diet Group	−12.0	−13.0	+1.0

TABLE X
Approximate Number of Calories Used Per Pound of Body Weight*

Activities	Cal/ hr./lb.	Activities	Cal/ hr./lb.
Daily Activities		**Sports, Recreation, Dance, Exercise**	
Carpentry or farm chores	1.55	Calisthenics	2.00
Class Work, lecture	0.67	Canadian Air Force	
Cleaning Windows	1.65	5BX & XBX Chart 1	3.31
Conversing	0.73	5BX & XBX Chart 2	4.16
Chopping Wood	2.92	5BX & XBX Charts 3 & 4	5.86
Driving	1.20	VBX Charts 5 & 6	6.64
Dressing/Showering	1.27	Dancing	
Eating	0.56	(Aerobic)	
Floor (mopping/sweeping)	1.83	light	1.87
Gardening	1.42	moderate	3.00
Gardening & Weeding	2.35	vigorous	4.40
Hoeing, Raking, Planting	1.88	(Modern)	
House Painting/Metal Work	1.40	moderate	1.67
Housework	1.62	vigorous	2.27
Kneeling	0.47	(Fox Trot)	1.78
Laying Brick	1.36	(Rhumba)	2.77
Making Bed	1.57	(Square)	2.74
Mowing Grass (power mower)	1.62	(Waltz)	2.05
(push mower)	1.78	Hill Climbing	3.90
Office Work	1.20	Motorcycling	1.45
Pick & Shovel Work	2.68	Mountain Climbing	4.02
Repairing Car (mechanic)	1.67	Walking	
Resting in Bed	0.48	2 mph	1.40
Sawing Wood	3.12	110-120 paces/min.	2.07
Shining Shoes	1.18	4½ mph	2.65
Shoveling Snow	3.11	Stair, up and back down	
Sleeping	0.46	1 step @ 25 trips/min.	2.73
Standing (no activity)	0.57	1 step @ 30 trips/min.	2.93
(light activity)	0.98	1 step @ 35 trips/min.	3.33
Watching T.V.	0.47	3 steps @ 12 trips/min.	3.19
Working in Yard	1.41	5 steps @ 10 trips/min.	4.00
Writing	0.73	7 steps @ 9 trips/min.	4.80

Adapted from Executive Fitness Newsletter, © 1975, 33 E. Minor Street, Emmaus, PA 18049.

The three groups lost about the same amount of weight; however, there was a difference in the body composition. The two exercise groups lost more fat than did the Diet Group as well as increasing their lean body tissue. The Diet Group lost both fat and *muscle*. The change in body composition exhibited by these women supports our contention that the most satisfactory method of weight control is a combination of diet and exercise. As one doctor puts it, "If 'homo laborans' becomes 'homo sedentarius' rather than 'homo sportius,' obesity will be an automatic consequence for many of our citizens."[2]

TABLE X—*Continued*

Sports Activities	Cal/hr./lb.	Sports Activities	Cal/hr./lb.
Archery	2.05	Sailing (calm water)	1.20
Badminton (mod.)	2.27	Skating (moderate)	2.27
(vigorous)	3.90	(vigorous)	4.10
Baseball (infield/outfield)	1.88	Skiing (downhill)	3.87
(pitching)	2.33	(level 5 mph)	4.68
Basketball (moderate)	2.82	Soccer	3.58
(vigorous)	3.96	Squash	4.15
(half court)	1.67	Swim (backstroke)	
Bicycling on level, 5.5 mph	2.00	20 yds./min.	1.55
13.0 mph	4.30	25 yds./min.	1.93
Bowling, non-stop	2.67	30 yds./min.	2.12
Canoeing, 4 mph	2.82	35 yds./min.	2.74
Fencing (moderate)	2.00	40 yds./min.	3.34
(vigorous)	4.10	(breaststroke)	
Football	3.32	20 yds./min.	1.93
Golf (twosome)	1.16	30 yds./min.	2.89
(foursome)	1.62	40 yds./min.	3.85
Handball (vigorous)	3.90	(butterfly)	4.68
Ping Pong	3.77	(Crawl)	
Rope Jumping 110 jumps/min.	3.86	20 yds./min.	1.93
120 jumps/min.	3.73	45 yds./min.	3.48
130 jumps/min.	3.46	50 yds./min.	4.25
Rowing (pleasure)	2.00	(sidestroke)	3.34
Rowing Machine or sculling		Tennis (moderate)	2.77
20 strokes/min.	5.46	(vigorous)	3.90
Running (level) 5.5 mph	4.30	Volleyball	2.33
7 mph	5.59	Water Skiing	3.12
9 mph	6.21	Weight Training	3.13
12 mph	7.87	Wrestling/Judo/Karate	5.13
(in place) 140 cts./min.	9.76		

Muscle tissue uses more calories than fat tissue. A lean person burns more calories than a fat person, and so finds it easier to stay slim. Calisthenics and weight training exercises which increase strength (and muscle mass) play as important a role in a flab control program as the high energy burning exercises.

One other aspect of exercise in weight and fat control is that *the increase in metabolism caused by the exercise may persist for hours after the activity has ceased, and thus continue to burn fat above that which was predicted.* For example, if you jog a mile, you might burn 125 calories, but you may actually burn an additional 25 or so calories in the hour following the run due to increased metabolism.

TABLE XI

The Caloric Cost of Running 1 1/2 Miles (2.4 km)*

Weight (lbs.)	Calories/minute								
	8	9	10	11	12	13	14	15	16
120	125	124	121	120	119	117	116	114	112
130	135	133	132	130	128	126	125	123	121
140	145	143	141	139	138	136	134	132	130
150	155	153	151	149	147	145	143	141	139
160	165	163	161	159	156	154	152	150	148
170	175	173	170	168	166	164	161	159	157
180	185	182	180	178	175	173	171	168	166
190	195	192	190	187	185	182	180	177	175
200	205	202	199	197	194	192	189	186	184
210	215	212	209	206	204	201	198	195	193
220	225	222	219	216	213	210	207	204	202

* Adapted from Harger, B. S. Miller, J. B. and Thomas, J. C., "The Caloric Cost of Running: Its Impact on Weight Reduction," *Journal of the American Medical Association,* 228:4, 1974.

Suggestions for Reducing

1. Consult your physician if you need to lose more than a few pounds. Weight reduction can actually be harmful.
2. Reduce caloric intake, but if you are not under a physician's supervision, do not reduce it below 1000-1200 calories. It is almost impossible to get an adequate supply of nutrients below this minimum. Do not waste your money on over-the-counter "diet pills."
3. Lose no more than one or two pounds per week unless you are under close medical supervision. After all, one pound a week is 52 pounds a year.
4. Combine your new eating habits with new exercise habits in a regimen you can live with for a lifetime. It must be practical and fit your likes and dislikes.
5. Do not expect a steady loss of weight; because the body temporarily adjusts the metabolism to try to maintain weight, and because there will be periods of temporary water retention, you may appear to gain or stop losing when you know that you should be losing. This is a most difficult period, but "Hang in there, baby!"; eventually you will see the rewards.
6. Weigh only once a week (same time of day, same scales, same clothing). Weight normally fluctuates about five pounds during the day and these temporary changes can be deceptive and discouraging.

Graph your weight change in half pound increments until you reach your goal. (see Chart IV A and IV B).

7. Diet and exercise with a friend or group who can reinforce you, share your victories and defeats, and help keep you working toward your goal.

8. Eat a balanced diet; cut down on (but do not eliminate) sweets, starches, fats, and oils. One doughnut less per day means a loss of two pounds per month; substituting a baked potato for fried potatoes once a week can eliminate four pounds a year; substituting a glass of skim milk for a glass of whole milk makes a difference of eight pounds per year. (see Table XII)

9. Avoid fad diets (see Chapter 5 on Quackery and Fallacies); there is no food or drug which will take off pounds. It's a million-dollar racket, so don't believe the ads. Low-calorie, liquid-formula diets, containing all essential nutrients, are not practical for long periods; however, they may be effective when used at the beginning of a diet regimen or as a replacement for a meal.

10. Reduce the size of the meal and add snacks for a fourth meal (but allow for the calories) if you feel hungry on a three-meal diet. Some studies show five small meals per day is better for reducing than three meals per day.

11. Eat breakfast to maintain your efficiency and help control your appetite at lunch. One-fourth of your daily caloric intake should be consumed at breakfast.

12. Eat many filling, low-calorie vegetables and keep animal protein high and carbohydrates low, but do not eat less than seventy grams of the latter. Research shows obese people overeat in the evenings—watch it!

13. Do not use the "rhythm method of girth control"—gaining and losing repeatedly may be more harmful than maintaining a steady overweight condition.

14. Record everything you eat, including the amount of the serving and the number of calories (See Charts VII and VIII in the Appendix). Eventually you will become "calorie wise" and learn to judge portions and calories. Refer to Tables XII, XIII, in this chapter for ways to save calories. Refer to Table XIV for a calorie counting guide.

Suggestions for Gaining

1. See your physician—you may need vitamin supplements or have other health problems needing attention.

2. Slow down—quit racing your engine; cut out the hurry by starting earlier. Plan ahead so you do not waste energy through inefficiency.

3. Get more rest and sleep; practice a conscious relaxation technique especially before meals (see Chapter 9).
4. Eat slowly and eat more; do not fill up on the bulky foods.
5. Have a well-balanced diet, but cut down on the protein and choose foods with more calories. Refer to Tables XII and XIII for ways to increase calories. Refer to Table XIV for help in finding high calorie foods.
6. Eat a hearty breakfast, and eat between meals if it does not dull your appetite. Five small meals a day might be more effective than three large meals.
7. Drink less fluid at meals and save room for the food.
8. Substitute milk for water when you are thirsty.
9. Do exercise for strength to increase the bulk of your muscles and perform rhythmical relaxation exercises.

How to Substitute Foods

The overweight person can save an enormous number of calories which will never be missed, and the underweight person can increase caloric intake without being gluttonous, by substituting food of equal nutritional value and taste and quality, but with a caloric value to fit their needs. Whether you are on a weight-gaining or weight-losing diet or just trying to maintain your weight, it pays to become calorie wise. In the sample meals (Table XII), the two extremes are compared to illustrate how the clever dieter can substitute foods.

TABLE XII

Sample Meals*

Breakfast			
High Cal	**Calories**	**Low Cal**	**Calories**
4 oz. orange juice	50	4 oz. orange juice	50
1 scrambled egg	120	1 boiled egg	78
2 slices bacon	100	1 slice bacon	50
2 slices white bread	126	2 slices gluten bread	70
2 pats butter	100	2 pats low cal margarine	34
2 cups coffee with 2 lumps		2 cups coffee with no-cal	
sugar and 2 tbsp. cream	220	sweetener and non-dairy cream	22
Total Calories	716	Total calories	304
Lunch			
Hamburger	350	Hamburger	350
1 slice apple pie	338	Low calorie pudding	123
1 glass (8 oz.) whole milk	165	1 glass (8 oz.) skim milk	80
Total Calories	853	Total Calories	553

*Used by permission of Pennwalt Prescription Products, *Are You Serious About Losing Weight*, Seventh Edition, 1973.

TABLE XII—*Continued*

Dinner

High Cal	Calories	Low Cal	Calories
½ glass (4 oz.) tomato juice	25	Consomme, 1 cup	10
6 oz. meat loaf	680	6 oz. club steak, broiled,	
with 4 tbsp. gravy		lean	320
(41 calories per tbsp.)	164	1 medium potato, baked	100
½ cup mashed potatoes	123	12 spears asparagus	40
½ cup green peas	72	2 pats low Calorie margarine	34
2 slices French bread	160	Hearts of lettuce	20
with 2 pats butter	100	with low calorie salad	
Tossed Salad	20	dressing	15
w/1½ tbsp. Roquefort		1 cup low Calorie whipped	
Cheese dressing (100		dessert	123
calories per tbsp.)	150	1 cup coffee with no-cal	
Iced plain layer cake	290	sweetener and non-dairy	
1 cup coffee with sugar		cream	11
(2 lumps) and cream			Total Calories 673
(2 tbsp.)	110		
	Total Calories 1894		

Snacks

High Cal	Calories	Low Cal	Calories
1 bottle cola beverage	105	Low calorie cola	2
1 custard (4 oz. cup)	205	2 low calorie cookies	50
1 cup coffee with sugar		1 cup coffee with no-cal	
(2 lumps) and cream		sweetener and non-dairy	
(2 tbsp.)	110	cream	11
1 small Danish pastry	140	2 low calorie cookies	50
	Total Calories 560		Total Calories 113

Total Calories for day 4023		Total Calories for day 1643	
		A saving of 2380 calories	

TABLE XIII

List of Foods Which Can Be Substituted for More or Less Calories*

High Cal	Calo-ries	Low Cal	Calo-ries	Differ-ence
		Beverages		
Milk (whole) 8 oz.	165	Milk (buttermilk or skim) 8 oz.	80	85
Prune juice, 8 oz.	170	Tomato Juice, 8 oz.	50	120
Soft drinks, 8 oz.	105	Diet soft drinks, 8 oz.	1	104
Coffee, cream, 2 tsp. sugar	110	Coffee (black with artificial sweetener)	0	110
Cocoa (all milk), 8 oz.	235	Cocoa (milk & water), 8 oz.	140	95
Chocolate malt, 8 oz.	500	Lemonade (sweetened), 8 oz.	100	400
Beer, 12 oz.	175	Lite Beer	100	75

*Used by permission of Pennwalt Prescription Products, *Are You Serious About Losing Weight,* Seventh Edition, 1973.

TABLE XIII—*Continued*

High Cal	Calo-ries	Low Cal	Calo-ries	Differ-ence
		Breakfast Foods		
Rice Flakes, 1 cup	110	Puffed Rice, 1 cup	50	60
Eggs (scrambled), 2	220	Eggs (boiled/poached) 2	160	60
		Butter and Cheese		
Butter on toast	170	Apple butter on toast	90	80
Cheese (Blue, Cheddar,		Cheese (cottage,		
Cream, Swiss), 1 oz.	105	uncreamed), 1 oz.	25	80
		Desserts		
Angel food cake, 2" piece	110	Cantaloupe melon, ½	40	70
Cheese cake, 2" piece	200	Watermelon, ½" slice		
Chocolate cake with icing,		(10" diam.)	60	140
2" piece	425	Sponge cake, 2" piece	120	305
Fruit cake, 2" piece	115	Grapes, 1 cup	65	50
Pound cake, 1 oz. piece	140	Plums, 2	50	90
Cupcake, white icing, 1	230	Plain cupcake, 1	115	115
Cookies, assorted		Vanilla wafer (dietetic),		
(3" diam.), 1	120	1	25	95
Ice cream, 4 oz.	150	Yogurt (flavored), 4 oz.	60	90
		Pies		
Apple, 1 piece (1/7 of a		Tangerine (fresh), 1	40	305
9" pie)	345			
Blueberry, 1 piece	290	Blueberries (frozen,		
		unsweetened), ½ cup	45	245
Cherry, 1 piece	355	Cherries (whole), ½ cup	40	315
Custard, 1 piece	280	Banana, small, 1	85	195
Lemon meringue, 1 piece	305	Lemon flavored gelatin,		
		½ cup	70	235
Peach, 1 piece	280	Peach, (whole), 1	35	245
Rhubarb, 1 piece	265	Grapefruit, ½	55	210
Pudding (flavored), ½ cup	140	Pudding (dietetic, non-		
		fat milk), ½ cup	60	80
		Fish and Fowl		
Tuna (canned), 3 oz.	165	Crabmeat (canned), 3 oz.	80	85
Oysters (fried), 6	400	Oysters (shell w/sauce) 6	100	300
Ocean perch (fried), 4 oz.	260	Bass, 4 oz.	105	155
Fish sticks, 5 sticks or 4 oz.	200	Swordfish (broiled), 3 oz.	140	60
Lobster meat, 4 oz. with		Lobster meat, 4 oz.		
2 tbsp. butter	300	with lemon	95	205
Duck (roasted), 3 oz.	310	Chicken (roasted), 3 oz.	160	150
		Meats		
Loin roast, 3 oz.	290	Pot roast (round), 3 oz.	160	130
Rump roast, 3 oz.	290	Rib roast, 3 oz.	200	90

TABLE XIII—*Continued*

High Cal	Calories	Low Cal	Calories	Difference
Swiss steak, 3½ oz.	300	Liver (fried), 2½ oz.	210	90
Hamburger (av. fat, broiled), 3 oz.	240	Hamburger (lean, broiled), 3 oz.	145	95
Porterhouse steak, 3 oz.	250	Club steak, 3 oz.	1606	90
Rib lamb chop (med.), 3 oz.	300	Veal chop (med.), 3 oz.	160	140
Pork chop (med.), 3 oz.	340	Veal chop (med.), 3 oz.	185	155
Pork roast, 3 oz.	310	Veal roast, 3 oz.	230	80
Pork sausage, 3 oz.	405	Ham (boiled, lean), 3 oz.	200	205

Potatoes

High Cal	Calories	Low Cal	Calories	Difference
Fried, 1 cup	480	Baked (2½″ diam.)	100	380
Mashed, 1 cup	245	Boiled (2½″ diam.)	100	140

Salads

High Cal	Calories	Low Cal	Calories	Difference
Chef salad with oil dressing, 1 tbsp.	180	Chef salad with dietetic dressing, 1 tbsp.	40	120
Chef salad with mayonnaise, 1 tbsp.	125	Chef salad with dietetic dressing, 1 tbsp.	40	85
Chef salad with Roquefort, Blue, Russian, French dressing, 1 tbsp.	105	Chef salad with dietetic dressing, 1 tbsp.	40	65

Sandwiches

High Cal	Calories	Low Cal	Calories	Difference
Club	375	Bacon and tomato (open)	200	175
Peanut butter and jelly	275	Egg salad (open)	165	110
Turkey with gravy, 3 tbsp.	520	Hamburger, lean, (open) 3 oz.	200	320

Snacks

High Cal	Calories	Low Cal	Calories	Difference
Fudge, 1 oz.	115	Vanilla wafers (dietetic), 2	50	65
Peanuts (salted), 1 oz.	170	Apple, 1	100	70
Peanuts (roasted), 1 cup shelled	1375	Grapes, 1 cup	65	1305
Potato chips, 10 med.	115	Pretzels, 10 small sticks	35	80
Chocolate, 1 oz. bar	145	Toasted marshmallows, 3	75	70

Soups

High Cal	Calories	Low Cal	Calories	Difference
Creamed, 1 cup	210	Chicken noodle, 1 cup	110	100
Bean, 1 cup	190	Beef noodle, 1 cup	110	80
Minestrone, 1 cup	105	Beef bouillon, 1 cup	10	95

Vegetables

High Cal	Calories	Low Cal	Calories	Difference
Baked beans, 1 cup	320	Green beans, 1 cup	30	290
Lima beans, 1 cup	160	Asparagus, 1 cup	30	130
Corn (canned), 1 cup	185	Cauliflower, 1 cup	30	155
Peas (canned), 1 cup	145	Peas (fresh), 1 cup	115	30
Winter squash, 1 cup	75	Summer squash, 1 cup	30	45
Succotash, 1 cup	260	Spinach, 1 cup	40	200

TABLE XIV

Calorie Guide to Common Foods

Beverages

Coffee (black)	3
Coke (12 oz.)	137
Hot chocolate, milk (1 cup)	247
Lemonade (1 cup)	100
Limeade, diluted to serve (1 cup)	110
Soda, fruit flavored (12 oz.)	161
Tea (clear)	3

Breads and Cereals

Bagel (1 half)	76
Biscuit (2" x 2")	135
Bread, Pita (1 oz.)	80
Bread, raisin (½" thick)	65
Bread, rye	55
Bread, white enriched (½" thick)	64
Bread, whole wheat (½" thick)	55
Bun (hamburger)	120
Cereals, cooked (½ cup)	80
Corn flakes (1 cup)	96
Corn Grits (1 cup)	125
Corn muffin (2½" diam.)	103
Crackers, graham (1 med.)	28
Crackers, soda (1 plain)	24
English muffin (1 half)	74
Macaroni, with cheese (1 cup)	464
Muffin, plain	135
Noodles (1 cup)	200
Oatmeal (1 cup)	150
Pancakes (1-4" diam.)	59
Pizza (1 section)	180
Popped corn (1 cup)	54
Potato chips (10 med.)	108
Pretzels (5 small sticks)	18
Rice (1 cup)	225
Roll, plain (1 med.)	118
Roll, sweet (1 med.)	178
Shredded wheat (1 med. biscuit)	79
Spaghetti, plain cooked (1 cup)	218
Tortilla (1 corn)	70
Waffle (4½" x 5")	216

Dairy Products

Butter, 1 pat (1½ tsp.)	50
Cheese, cheddar (1 oz.)	113
Cheese, cottage (1 cup)	270
Cheese, cream (1 oz.)	106
Cheese, Parmesan (1 tbsp.)	29
Cheese, Swiss natural (1 oz.)	105
Cream, sour (1 tbsp.)	31
Dairy Queen Cone (med.)	335
Frozen custard (1 cup)	375
Frozen yogurt, vanilla (1 cup)	180

Ice cream, plain (prem.) (1 cup)	350
Ice cream soda, choc. (large glass)	455
Ice milk (1 cup)	184
Ices (1 cup)	177
Milk, chocolate (1 cup)	185
Milk, half-and-half (1 tbsp.)	20
Milk, malted (1 cup)	281
Milk, skim (1 cup)	88
Milk, skim dry (1 tbsp.)	28
Milk, whole (1 cup)	166
Sherbert (1 cup)	270
Whipped topping (1 tbsp.)	14
Yogurt (1 cup)	150

Desserts and Sweets

Cake, angel (2" wedge)	108
Cake, chocolate (2" x 3" x 1")	150
Cake, plain (3" x 2½")	180
Chocolate, bar	200-300
Chocolate, bitter (1 oz.)	142
Chocolate, sweet (1 oz.)	133
Chocolate, syrup (1 tbsp.)	42
Cocoa (1 tbsp.)	21
Cookies, plain (1 med.)	75
Custard, baked (1 cup)	283
Doughnut (1 large)	250
Gelatin, dessert (1 cup)	155
Gelatin, with fruit (1 cup)	170
Gingerbread (2" x 2" x 2")	180
Jams, jellies (1 tbsp.)	55
Pie, apple (1/7 of 9" pie)	345
Pie, cherry (1/7 of 9" pie)	355
Pie, chocolate (1/7 of 9" pie)	360
Pie, coconut (1/7 of 9" pie)	266
Pie, lemon meringue (1/7 of 9" pie)	302
Sugar, granulated (1 tsp.)	27
Syrup, table (1 tbsp.)	57

Fruit

Apple, fresh (med.)	76
Applesauce, unsweetened (1 cup)	184
Avocado, raw (½ peeled)	279
Banana, fresh (med.)	88
Cantaloupe, raw (½, 5" diam.)	60
Cherries (10 sweet)	50
Cranberry sauce, unsweetened (1 tbsp.)	25
Fruit cocktail, canned (1 cup)	170
Grapefruit, fresh (½)	60
Grapefruit, juice, raw (1 cup)	95
Grape juice, bottled (½ cup)	80
Grapes (20-25)	75
Nectarine (1 med.)	88

Note: For a complete listing of foods, the reader is referred to: *Nutritive Value of Foods*, U.S. Department of Agriculture, Washington, D.C., Home and Gardens Bulletin, No. 72. (Available in most libraries, university bookstores, and Home Economics departments).

TABLE XIV—*Continued*

Olives, green (10)	72
Olives, ripe (10)	105
Orange, fresh (med.)	60
Orange juice, frozen diluted (1 cup)	110
Peach, fresh (med.)	46
Peach, canned in syrup (2 halves)	79
Pear, fresh (med.)	95
Pears, canned in syrup (2 halves)	79
Pineapple, crushed in syrup (1 cup)	204
Pineapple (½ cup fresh)	50
Prune juice (1 cup)	170
Raisins, dry (1 tbsp.)	26
Strawberries, fresh (1 cup)	54
Strawberries, frozen (3 oz.)	90
Tangerine (2½″ diam.)	40
Watermelon, wedge (4″ x 8″)	120

Meat, Fish, Eggs

Bacon, drained (2 slices)	97
Bacon, Canadian (1 oz.)	62
Beef, hamburger chuck (3 oz.)	316
Beef, pot pie	560
Beef steak, sirloin or T-bone (3 oz.)	257
Beef and vegetable stew (1 cup)	185
Chicken, fried breast (8 oz.)	210
Chicken, fried (1 leg and thigh)	305
Chicken, roasted breast (2 slices)	100
Chili, without beans (1 cup)	510
Chili, with beans (1 cup)	335
Egg, boiled	77
Egg, fried	125
Egg, scrambled	100
Fish and Chips (2 pcs. fish; 4 oz. chips)	275
Fish, broiled (3″ x 3″ x½″)	112
Fish stick	40
Frankfurter, boiled	124
Ham (4″ x 4″)	338
Lamb (3 oz. roast, lean)	158
Liver (3″ x 3″)	150
Luncheon meat (2 oz.)	135
Pork chop, loin (3″ x 5″)	284
Salmon, canned (1 cup)	145
Sausage, pork (4 oz.)	510
Shrimp, canned (3 oz.)	108
Tuna, canned (½ cup)	185
Veal, cutlet (3″ x 4″)	175

Nuts and Seeds

Cashews (1 cup)	770
Coconut (1 cup)	450
Peanut butter (1 tbsp.)	92
Peanuts, roasted, no skin (1 cup)	805
Pecans (1 cup)	752
Sunflower seeds, (1 tbsp.)	50

Sandwiches
(2 slices of bread—plain)

Bologna	214
Cheeseburger (small McDonald)	300
Chicken salad	185
Egg salad	240
Fish Filet (McDonald's)	400
Ham	360
Ham and cheese	360
Hamburger (small McDonald's)	260
Hamburger, Burger King Whopper	600
Hamburger, Big Mac	550
Hamburger, McDonald's Quarter Pounder	420
Peanut butter	250
Roast Beef (Arby's Regular)	425

Sauces, Fats, Oils

Catsup, tomato (1 tbsp.)	17
Chili sauce (1 tbsp.)	17
French dressing (1 tbsp.)	59
Margarine (1 pat)	50
Mayonnaise (1 tbsp.)	92
Mayonnaise-type (1 tbsp.)	65
Vegetable, sunflower, safflower oils (1 tbsp.)	120

Soup, Ready to Serve

Bean (1 cup)	190
Beef noodle	100
Cream	200
Tomato	90
Vegetable	80

Vegetables

Alfalfa sprouts (½ cup)	19
Asparagus (6 spears)	22
Bean sprouts (1 cup)	37
Beans, green (1 cup)	27
Beans, lima (1 cup)	152
Beans, navy (1 cup)	642
Beans, pork and molasses (1 cup)	325
Broccoli, fresh cooked (1 cup)	60
Cabbage, cooked (1 cup)	40
Cauliflower (1 cup)	25
Carrot, raw (med.)	21
Carrots, canned (1 cup)	44
Celery, diced raw (1 cup)	20
Coleslaw (1 cup)	102
Corn, sweet, canned (1 cup)	140
Corn, sweet (med. ear)	84
Cucumber, raw (6 slices)	6
Lettuce (2 large leaves)	7
Mushrooms, canned (1 cup)	28
Onions, french fried (10 rings)	75
Onions, raw (med.)	25

TABLE XIV—*Continued*

Peas, field (½ cup)	90	Sauerkraut, drained (1 cup)	32
Peas, green (1 cup)	145	Spinach, fresh, cooked (1 cup)	46
Pickles, dill (med.)	15	Squash, summer (1 cup)	30
Pickles, sweet (med.)	22	Sweet pepper (med.)	15
Potato, baked (med.)	97	Sweet potato, candied (small)	314
Potato, french fried (8 stick)	155	Tomato, cooked (1 cup)	50
Potato, mashed (1 cup)	185	Tomato, raw (med)	30
Radish, raw (small)	1		

References

1. M. B. Zuti, "Effects of Diet and Exercise on Body Composition of Adult Women During Weight Reduction," doctoral dissertation, Kent State University, 1972, as reported in *Physical Fitness Research Digest*, President's Council on Physical Fitness, Washington, D.C., Series 5, No. 2 (April, 1975).
2. Division of Chronic Diseases, Heart Disease Control Program, *Obesity and Health* (Washington: Public Health Service, U.S. Department of Health, Education and Welfare), 43.

Quackery and Fallacies

5

Quacks and hucksters are bilking the public of millions of dollars each year on gadgets, so-called health foods, diets, and pills which are useless and sometimes even harmful. Radio, television, newspapers, and books frequently carry false or misleading advertisements and incorrect information about exercise and weight control. Surveys show that a large percentage of people believe that if something is "in print" or is said "on the air," then it must be true. Unfortunately, this is not the case because our laws and means of enforcing them are inadequate to prevent most of the hoaxes perpetrated on the consumer. The only real protection is the educated consumer; to that end, this brief expose is dedicated.

Fad Diets

There are hundreds of fad diets, usually used to sell books or special ingredients in the diet. Typically they manipulate protein, fat, and carbohydrates so that one or two components are markedly increased while the other(s) is drastically decreased or eliminated. The dangers in these are as follows.

No or Low Fat Diet—may lead to hunger, irritability, dry skin and scalp, stiff joints, constipation, poor concentration, general unhealthiness.

High Fat Diet (usually combined with high protein and low carbohydrate)—may cause diarrhea, loss of nutrients and electrolytes, and high cholesterol levels (this may cause heart disease).

No or Low Carbohydrate (usually combined with high protein and high fat)—may cause excessive retention of uric acid, gout, kidney problems, complications for the diabetic or pregnant woman, hypoglycemia, dizziness, weakness, dehydration, nausea, irritability.

No or Low Protein—may result in weakness, loss of muscle and organ tissues; it is dangerous to fall below 70 grams.

No juggling of the above nutrients is effective in making you lose weight or gain weight or improve your sex life. Calories do count. Whether you count them or follow a pre-counted diet, it is the number of calories rather than the source of the calories which determines weight loss/gain.

Diet Foods and Supplements

All foods contain calories. There is *no* such thing as a reducing food, negative calorie food, or food with special ability to burn off fat. Grapefruit is not a yellow spark-plug. Protein supplements will *not* make you lose weight. A liquid protein diet is not a safe way to reduce. It may cause an irregular heart beat which can be fatal. Safflower oil does *not* loosen long-stored fat. Vinegar, vitamin B_6 and Lecithin have *no* beneficial properties in a weight or fat loss program. Diet beer, diet chocolate pudding, diet bars, etc., etc., contain calories, and eaten in enough quantity can make you gain. Water has *no* calories and is *not* a food, but many people on a water diet think that the eight glasses of water per day make the diet successful. Sunflower seed oil is no lower in calories or cholesterol than are other vegetable oils. Everyone does not need to take vitamin and mineral supplements. It is possible to "O.D." on vitamins. Prolonged overdosing of vitamin C, for example, can cause kidney stones, diarrhea, and heart burn. Sudden withdrawal can cause scurvy-like symptoms. Other vitamins and supplements similarly cause toxicity when abused.

Reducing Drugs

Prescription Drugs

In the 1950s-60s, obesity clinics freely prescribed a potent combination of drugs known as "Rainbow Pills" which included amphetamines, barbiturates, thyroid, digitalis, diuretics, laxatives, antispasmodics, and hypotensive agents. These resulted in so many cases of deafness, blindness, paralysis, and even death that the government has drastically limited the writing of such prescriptions. Besides being dangerous in combinations, many of them are addictive, and all merely serve as crutches, but fail to change the eating patterns of the patients.

Over-the-Counter Drugs

There are probably a thousand non-prescription drugs available, all of which are ineffective; as quickly as the Food and Drug Administration removes them from the market, they reappear under a new name. There are bulk producers (such as glucomanan) which it is claimed will fill the stomach and reduce hunger pains, but which actually work only in the intestines and have no effect on appetite. There are appetite depressants, such as those containing phenylpropanolamine (p.p.a. or propradine). In spite of the fact that the F.D.A. approved this drug studies show it to be ineffective in the recommended doses and if larger doses are taken, especially by those with heart disease, thyroid problems, high blood pressure, and diabetes, it may be dangerous. Starch blockers are believed to be ineffective as well as unsafe.

Lotions, Creams, Diet Candy, Diet Chewing Gum and Diet Cigarettes

These are equally ineffective in a weight or girth control program. There is nothing known to modern science which is safe and effective for you to rub on, drink, chew, or smoke to lose weight. Accustaple (staples in the ears) has not been proven effective. Injections of *HCG* lack scientific evidence of effectiveness. Generally, one may assume that anyone who claims to have a quick and easy cure is a quack.

Gadgets and Gimmicks

Passive Exercise Machines

Passive exercise, in which a machine or another person moves your body with little or no effort on your part, is useless for weight or girth reduction. Examples of some of these ineffective devices include:

Rollers—whether hand-held or motor driven, these wooden or metal cylinders have no effect on weight, shape, or fat when rolled up and down on the body part.

Vibrating Belts, Tables, and Pillows—these gadgets which shake the person or body part do not "break-up fatty deposits," improve posture, or take off inches.

Motor Driven Bicycles and Rowing Machines—these devices move the arms and legs of the rider who sits passively. They contribute nothing to the fitness or girth control of the normal person.

Massage—whether given by a mechanical device or by a masseur, this manipulation of the tissues is passive. It may have some therapeutic benefits but it does not aid in improving fitness or figure/physique.

Sauna, Steam, and Whirlpool Baths

Dry sauna, wet sauna, steam baths, whirlpool baths, hot tubs, and other forms of applying heat and water are claimed by their proponents to do everything from melting off pounds to curing bronchitis, improving complexion, and "ridding the body of toxins and poisons." One sauna manufacturer even claims his device cures cancer! The truth is, they do none of these things. Some people enjoy the largely psychological effect of the baths and find them relaxing. Persons with chronic arthritis, sprains, bruises, and muscle soreness may find temporary relief induced by the heat; but the same beneficial effects can be obtained by sitting in a tub of hot water at home. The heat in the baths will cause the body to perspire and lose body fluids (dehydrate). Dehydration causes a temporary loss of weight until the water is replaced by normal eating and drinking. The baths do not melt off fat.

Sauna and steam baths can be dangerous for the elderly, or for bathers suffering from diabetes, heart trouble, and high blood pressure, as well as those under the influence of hypnotics, narcotics, or tranquilizers. This is *not* a good way to get rid of a hangover. Prolonged exposure can result in severe dehydration, causing not only water loss but also a deprivation of mineral salts. This can lead to heat stroke and, eventually, to brain damage and death.

Non-Porous Garments

"Melts pounds away as you work or play," says the advertisement for non-porous garments such as sauna suits (jeans, shorts, belts, sleepwear, and girdles). These garments have been on the market for a number of years under a variety of trade names. They are made of material (such as rubber) which is non-porous and holds in body heat, causing perspiration and/or they fit tightly and may even be inflatable. The latter varieties of air belts and shorts are like plastic innertubes which serve as constricting bands as well as non-porous garments.

Perspiration causes dehydration and a temporary weight loss of body fluids (not a fat loss). Constricting bands can squeeze the superficial fluids into deeper tissues of the body and cause a temporary indentation and decrease in girth just as a tight watch band leaves an indentation on the wrist. These bands do not squeeze out fat and have no value. They may even cause medical problems by interfering with blood flow in the veins from the lower extremities back to the heart.

Weighted Belts

Belts containing lead granules and weighing 6 to 9 pounds have been advertised to be worn under clothing throughout the day for weight loss, waist slimming, and physical fitness. One study showed it would take a 200 pound man 45 days to burn enough calories to lose 1 pound. These belts not only have been found to be ineffective, but they were ordered off the market by the government because they resulted in injuries to the lower back and caused joint strain.

Muscle Stimulators

A variety of electronic "effortless exercise" devices have been on the market since the 1930s, which claim to "tone flabby muscles" and cause a girth reduction. These are muscle stimulators, similar to those used in hospital physical therapy departments, which send an electric current into the muscle, causing it to contract involuntarily. Some of these devices might actually be effective, but could be very dangerous in the hands of the public. Government agencies have attempted to remove some of these machines from the market because they have been found to aggravate many medical conditions.

Bust Developers

Charlatans have offered a variety of gimmicks purported to enlarge the female breasts—lotions, hormone creams, suction pumps, water massage, electrical muscle stimulators, and exercise devices. The breasts, of course, are mammary glands composed largely of fatty tissue and suspended by ligaments. They are not muscles and can not be exercised or stimulated to contract. The breast lies on top of the pectoralis major, a large muscle on the chest; when the pectoral muscle is strengthened it increases in mass (hypertrophy), and causes an increase in the chest girth; there is no way to increase the size of the breasts other than augmentation surgery (silicon transplants) or silicon injections. The latter are considered unsafe.

Cellulite

One of the more recent frauds is the claim that 8 out of 10 women have a "fat-gone-wrong" called cellulite (pronounced sell-u-leet) that will not respond to diet and exercise. Presumably, it looks dimpled like orange peeling and needs special treatment. This rip-off is used to sell books and strange treatments such as a stream of hot air directed on a body part while an automated suction massage machine works on the fat. This is bunk! The word *cellulite* is not likely to be found in medical books; it refers to ordinary superficial adipose tissue—fat, which may or may not look like orange peel, but which will be lost only when there is a calorie deficit.

Figure Wrapping

Some reducing salons and mail order establishments claim you can lose from 4 to 12 inches in one treatment, with no diet and no exercise. The treatment consists of a hot shower, followed by being wrapped like a mummy in linen bandages dipped in a "magic solution"; then an hour of waiting encased in a sauna suit in a cold room. The solutions vary, but are apt to be epsom salts (magnesium sulfate and aluminum sulfate), glycerin and herbs and spices. There is a slight, temporary decrease in girth measurements due to the constricting pressure squeezing body fluids to deeper tissues and the hypertonic effect of the solution which tends to dehydrate the superficial tissues. The cold room may produce further body shrinkage from hypothermia, as the blood vessels constrict to conserve heat. These effects are *temporary* and will disappear in a few hours. The treatment is *dangerous,* has caused the death of at least one woman, and can be harmful to those with heart or circulatory problems, varicose veins, phlebitis, or kidney trouble.

Reducing Salons, Health Clubs, Spas

The typical establishment is a highly commercial business more interested in making a profit than in the welfare of the client. Its personnel are generally not qualified and rarely have degrees or certificates in physical therapy, physical education, or corrective therapy. Most are hired for their nice appearance and are trained on the job in a few short weeks. They are not qualified to diagnose and prescribe for health, figure/physique, or fitness problems. Most establishments offer all the passive exercise gimmicks and baths, and some include figure wrapping and the prescription of fad diets. Most provide active exercise programs and weight lifting equipment, also, but they rarely give training for cardiovascular endurance. Many of the treatment claims are false or misleading, and some of their programs can be harmful.

They do offer facilities and equipment and a pleasant place to meet and exercise with your friends (at a price), but as a general rule, it would be better to investigate programs offered by the local YMCA-YWCA, Parks and Recreation Departments, University, and Community Colleges. There are some good commercial fitness centers with qualified personnel (with degrees in physical education, corrective therapy, physical therapy or exercise physiology). Diet clubs such as Tops and Weight Watchers are also reputable, but you would need to provide your own exercise program if you joined one of these.

Fallacies and Misconceptions

There are a number of fallacies and misconceptions in the weight and fatness control and physical fitness areas. Some of these are included below along with brief statements regarding the true facts.

Fallacy: *Obesity is caused by gluttony.*

Chapter 4 briefly described some of the causes of obesity, including the summary statement that the overweight (fat) person consumes more calories than are burned. This is a correct concept, but it often is misinterpreted to mean that fat people are gluttons. Most overweight is of the "creeping" kind caused by a gradual slow-down in activity and metabolism as we get older, without an accompanying decrease in our caloric consumption. There are some gluttons among the obese, but there are many more who eat less than their non-fat counterparts. When they say, "But I hardly eat enough to keep a bird alive," for some, it may be true. Several studies of boys and girls have shown that the fat ones ate less than their normal weight peers, but were less active physically. Similar studies on adults and animals confirm that inactivity contributes to much obesity.

Fallacy: *Exercise increases the appetite and therefore should be avoided by a person trying to reduce.*

Both animal and human studies carried out by nutritionists refute this idea. The sedentary person who begins an exercise program will usually take in more food than is burned in activity and will gain weight. The normally active person will tend to increase food intake, but it will be balanced by the activity output so that no weight is gained. The person who exercises to exhaustion will tend to lose both appetite and weight.

Fallacy: *Exercising the spot where fat is deposited will make the fat come off of that spot.*

As previously mentioned, the location of fat deposits is controlled genetically and differs somewhat from person to person. If too much of it is deposited in a spot where we do not want it, we call it a "trouble spot" and wish we could get rid of it or shift it to areas where we need more padding. The "spot exercise" fallacy assumes, for example, that if you have "pones" (fat deposits) on the side of your hips, exercising the muscles underlying that fat will make it go away. Some not very scientific observations in the late 1800s are probably responsible for this misconception but more recent, careful investigations show that when we exercise, fuel comes from the bloodstream and the body, acting as a composite unit, mobilizes fat from all over the body. The contracting muscle has no direct connection with the overlying adipose layer and does not get its energy from that particular piece of blubber.

General exercises are just as effective as "spot exercises" to remove fat. Any exercise burns calories (fat) and the fat comes from all over the body. One study showed that there is a tendency to lose more fat from the areas that are fattest. When someone says, "When I lose weight, I lose it in the wrong places; I always lose it from my face where I need it least," the truth of the matter is, they probably lose it from all over, but a fourth of an inch is more noticeable when lost from the face than it is when lost from the waist or hips. Local exercises are good to develop strength and endurance in specific muscle groups and do burn calories; *they do not selectively reduce fat deposits.*

Fallacy: *Bumping fat body parts against the floor or wall will help reduce the fat.*

Bumping, thumping, massaging, rolling, vibrating, and shaking body parts are forms of passive exercise. To be useful for girth reduction, an exercise must make the muscle contract. When it does so, calories are burned and fat is mobilized. In addition, if an exercise is at the threshold of training, the muscle will get stronger and will experience hypertrophy (increase in size). Muscle tissue is more compact than fat. A pound of fat takes up more room than a pound of muscle, so that increasing lean body mass while decreasing fat means a loss in inches if weight remains constant. Finally, strong, firm muscles can hold the body parts in positions of good posture, to give a slimmer appearance. Weak muscles in any area— hips, thighs, waist, arms—lead to a conditon called flabbiness, and strengthening those specific muscles can change the body contour.

Fallacy: *Exercise can get rid of wrinkles and sagging skin.*

There is a phenomenon experienced with the aging process called "atrophy," in which body tissues begin to deteriorate. Proper exercise tends to delay the process in some tissues, but there is one physique problem that can not be altered by exercise. Sometimes around middle age, the subcutaneous tissues (those just under the skin) begin to atrophy noticeably and the skin loses its elasticity and seems to hang in flaps. It is what makes the jaw line sag and jowls and wrinkles develop. Other common cosmetic problems are the flapping of the backs of the upper arms and the sagging of the seat. Face lifts and other plastic surgery procedures can remove these tell-tale marks of aging, but exercise is very limited in its effectiveness. It can not put elasticity back into the skin that has lost it nor build up atrophied subcutaneous tissues. It can not remove wrinkles nor get rid of stretch marks nor skin flaps. Exercise can firm up (strengthen) flabby muscles and add a little bulk to fill out sagging skin. And it can help improve fitness and health of the aging person so that they feel and act younger.

Posture: Static and Dynamic

6

For the truth about your posture—ask your mirror; or better yet, have someone take a posture picture of you. On Chart IX in the Appendix, you will find places to attach your posture pictures. Underneath the pictures, your instructor can check your postural defects and give you an overall rating of them. Most of these defects are discussed in this unit.

The position in which you hold your body while lying, sitting, standing, or moving is called *posture*. Three things contribute to better posture and good health: a sufficient amount of sleep, proper exercise, and a balanced diet.

Some of the factors conducive to poor posture are fatigue, obesity, self consciousness (e.g., disguising one's height by slumping), occupational conditions, (e.g., mail carrier with a heavy mail bag), and faulty habits. Bending over a low sink while washing dishes (working surfaces should be at elbow height), and watching TV or studying while sitting in a poor position are examples of faulty postural habits.

Postural Defects

1. **Round Shoulders**—Tips of the shoulders held forward. (This is usually accompanied by a forward head, sunken chest, and protruding scapulae.)
2. **Scoliosis**—Lateral curvature of the spine. This may be a very serious deformity and it requires referral to a physician. See illustration on p. 89.
3. **Lordosis**—Increased hyper-extension in the lumbar region ("sway back").
4. **Abdominal Ptosis**—Protruding abdomen (often accompanies lordosis).
5. **Kyphosis**—Round upper back ("hump back").
6. **Flat Back**—Decreased spinal curvature or not enough curve, especially in the lower back.

7. **Hyperextended Knees**—Knees thrown back in a locked position. This habit often causes lordosis.
8. **Protruding Scapulae**—Protruding shoulder blades, or "wings."
9. **Body Lean**—A body shift from the ankles, either too far forward or backward.
10. **Forward Head**—Head thrust forward ("poke neck").
11. **Sunken Chest**—Low or depressed chest.
12. **Fatique Slump**—Hips thrust forward; trunk leaning backward; spinal flexion extends into lumbar region, with hyper-extension at the sacro-iliac joint.

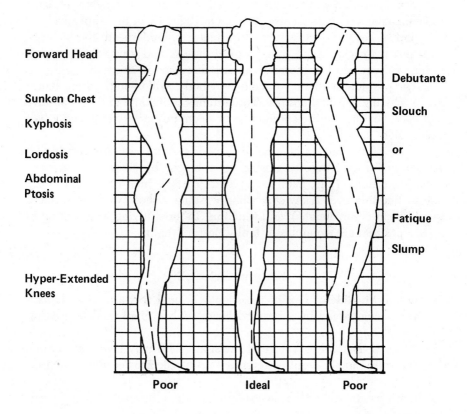

Forward Head

Sunken Chest

Kyphosis

Lordosis

Abdominal Ptosis

Hyper-Extended Knees

Debutante

Slouch

or

Fatique

Slump

Poor   Ideal   Poor

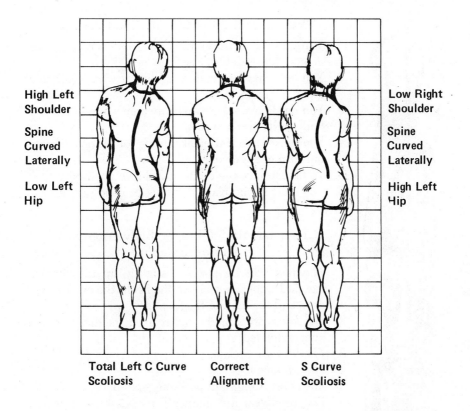

High Left
Shoulder

Spine
Curved
Laterally

Low Left
Hip

Low Right
Shoulder

Spine
Curved
Laterally

High Left
Hip

Total Left C Curve   Correct   S Curve
Scoliosis   Alignment Scoliosis

Why Have Good Posture

Perhaps the most obvious reason for obtaining good posture is that you will look better—and everyone wants to make a good *appearance.* Remember, the first impression you make upon a stranger is visual! In addition, *your clothes will probably fit better;* therefore, you will not have to wear loosely fitted clothes just to hide the "real you." Another reason for having good posture is that you will be more *efficient,* since joints, ligaments, and muscles will not be strained by poor posture and the range of movement will be greater. Finally, certain postural faults are linked to poor health. Lordosis probably makes one more susceptible to backache and dysmenorrhea; round shoulders and sunken chest may impair respiratory capacity; and head forward may lead to a variety of aches in the head, face, neck, and arms. Scoliosis will result in serious deformity if not treated early and a painful back will result.

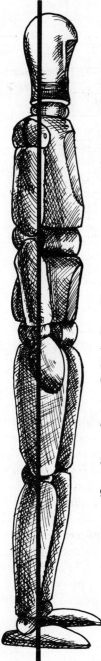

Prerequisites for Achieving Good Posture

1. You must be born with a body free from congenital or hereditary deformities.
2. You must have an understanding of what constitutes good posture.
3. You must have a kinesthetic awareness of where your body parts are in space.
4. You must have sufficient muscle tonus for maintaining correct alignment.
5. You must have the desire to achieve good posture.
6. You must be motivated to practice good posture.

Characteristics of Proper Body Alignment During Standing

1. *The feet* will be parallel, slightly apart, with the weight balanced evenly on the heels, the outside borders, and the balls of the feet.
2. *The knees* are straight and relaxed—neither bent nor hyperextended.
3. *The hips* are tucked.
4. *The abdomen* is flat.
5. *The chest* is high but not exaggerated.
6. *The shoulders* are neither forward, backward, nor elevated, but free and easy, with the shoulder blades flat.
7. *The head* is centered over the trunk, with the *chin* level and the *ears* in line with the tips of the shoulders.
8. *The arms* hang relaxed, with the palms of the hands facing the sides of the body.
9. *The back* is neither too flat nor too curved.

If each body segment is balanced, a vertical line should extend from behind the ear, through the center of the shoulder and hip, behind the kneecap, and just in front of the ankle. Whenever one part moves out of line, the center of gravity shifts in the direction of movement of that segment, and another segment must adjust in the opposite direction to bring the center of gravity back over the base. A body is balanced when its center of gravity is over its supporting base. When wearing high heeled shoes or boots, the center of gravity should be adjusted at the ankles without disturbing the alignment of the various segments. If the backward adjustment is made at the waist, as is frequently the case, the entire alignment is affected and strain is felt in the lower back. The same principle is true in counterbalancing the added weight in pregnancy or when carrying an object.

Muscles work in pairs, and both must be exercised in order not to have postural faults. For example, strengthening the chest muscles could cause round shoulders and sunken chest unless the upper back muscles are also strengthened.

If your body segments are not in alignment, you may need to strengthen weak muscle groups and stretch tight or short muscle groups by the use of special exercise.

The maintenance of proper posture depends upon sufficient muscular endurance. Muscular endurance is the ability of a muscle to perform work for a sustained period. Muscles which fatigue easily will be unable to maintain correct body alignment.

Most of us need reminders to aid us in achieving good posture. These key words might be helpful.

1. *Stand tall.*   3. *Walk tall.*
2. *Sit tall.*   4. *Think tall.*

Sitting and Rising

Much of your day is spent, sitting. You sit to eat, study, work, and socialize. You sit in class, in a theater, in church, and at an athletic event. Not only should your sitting posture be good, but the act of getting into and out of the seated position should be performed gracefully and efficiently.

Sitting In and Rising from a Chair

As you enter a room, choose the chair best suited to you. Ideally, a chair should have arms, be low enough to allow you to place your feet

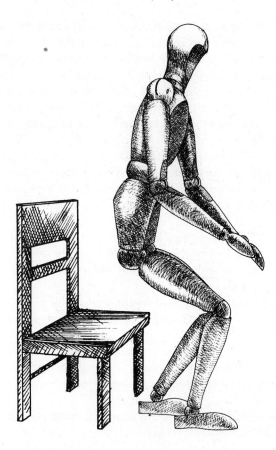

on the floor while keeping your knees above hip level, and be shallow enough for your back to be placed against the chair back.

Approach the chair at a slight angle from the right or left, and touch the center front of the chair with the calf of your leg as you turn your back to it. The foot nearest the chair should be well under it, with your weight on both feet. Keep your neck and head in line with your trunk and your trunk erect, with the hips tucked under as you bend at the hips and knees and incline your body slightly forward. Shift your body weight to your rear foot, as your body is lowered into the chair, by using the leg muscles. Keep your pelvis under your trunk, your feet under your pelvis, and transfer the body weight gradually and smoothly.

Certain types of chairs present problems. More muscular effort is needed if the seat is low. If the seat is deep, the hands may be placed on the chair arms to help retain balance, but try to avoid using the arms to lower your body.

Sit on the whole chair—if a "scoot" is necessary, try to move back in one attempt. Sit on the two knob-like pelvic bones (tuberosities of the ischia); hold the head and chest erect, with the abdomen in; lean against the back rest; and relax your shoulders. Women, should cross their legs above the knee or at the ankle. Some women prefer to place the heel of one foot against the instep of the other foot, keeping the knees together.

To rise, simply reverse the sitting procedure. If it is necessary to "scoot" forward, try to do it in one attempt. Place one foot as far back under the chair as possible. Lean slightly forward from the hips, keeping your hips tucked under and your chest and head erect. Push up by extending the knee of the rear foot as you shift your weight from the rear foot to the front foot. Use your thigh muscles to "press into the floor" by pushing on your heels. Your hands may be placed on the arms of the chair to help you retain your balance, but do not push up with them.

Walking

You should walk the way you stand—with a well-balanced, relaxed, and poised body alignment. The purpose in walking is to move forward; therefore, there should be no wasted motion in the lateral plane. Limit the motion to arms and legs with a minimum of trunk movement.

Stand in your best posture. Swing your leg straight ahead, keeping your knee flexed, with the major movement flowing from the hip. Point your toes straight ahead. Place the heel of your foot very lightly on the floor; transfer your weight to the outer border and then the ball; "feel" the floor with your toes; and then push off with the big toe. Move the feet on parallel tracks, about two inches apart. Stride length will vary with the type of dress, leg length, and speed of your gait; but in general, it will be approximately the length of your foot. Let your arms swing freely and easily from the shoulder joint in opposition to your leg movements. The length of the swing depends on the length of the stride—just enough to keep your chest facing forward. The palm of your hand should face your leg, with finger tips just brushing lightly in passing.

Since there is no one best standing posture, there is no one best walking gait. Body structures and personalities vary and are expressed in an individual's walk. However, wide variation may need to be modified.

Stair Climbing

Good body mechanics in ascending and descending stairs should be considered from the standpoints of safety, efficiency, and appearance.

Several factors are important in regard to safety. Place your entire foot on the step to prevent arch strain and to help retain balance. Many steps are narrow, so it may be necessary to turn the body slightly sideways in order to place the entire foot on the tread. Glance occasionally at several steps ahead of you; however, do not look at your feet. You should use the handrail to help retain balance by sliding the hand lightly along the rail.

When ascending stairs, the body should be lifted forward and upward with the leg of your *forward* foot. The knee is bent as your foot is placed on the step, and is extended with the strong thigh (quadriceps) muscles as the weight is transferred to the lead foot. When descending, the knee is bent, and the body weight is supported by the strong thigh muscles (again using the quadriceps) of the *rear* leg as the weight is transferred to the lead foot.

Your posture should be erect. Carry your head and chest high, and avoid pushing the hips backward when taking each step. Watch where you are going by occasionally focusing your eyes on the steps ahead without jutting your head forward. Move your body smoothly and steadily in a gliding manner. A jerky bounce can be avoided by using the knees as "shock absorbers," keeping them slightly bent and not straightening them on every step.

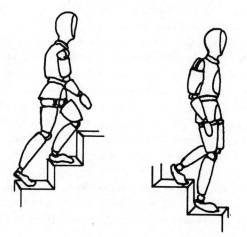

Selected Exercises for Postural Faults

Abdominal Ptosis (These exercises are also good for lordosis.)

Cat-Backs (strengthens abdominals). On hands and knees permit the abdominals "to droop" and the back to sway. Then flatten the abdomen by "pulling it in," and "hump" the back, holding for a count of five. Relax for five counts and repeat five times.

Pelvic Tilt (strengthens abdominals). An isometric exercise done in a supine position, with the knees bent and slightly apart. Press the spine down on the floor and hold it while tightening the abdominals and gluteals. Hold for ten counts, and relax. Repeat five times.

Sit-ups (strengthens abdominals). Refer to Chapter 1 "Tests for Physical Fitness." When performed for the purpose of abdominal strengthening, it is best to leave the feet free and unsupported. This helps to insure that the proper muscles are performing the work and avoids strain on the back.

Lordosis

Wall Exercise (strengthens abdominals and stretches the lower back). Stand with your back to the wall and the heels an inch from the wall. Flatten the lower back against the wall and walk away maintaining the flattened back. Return to the wall and check to see if you have kept that position.

Knee Raise (stretches lower back). Lie in supine position. Bend one knee and bring it to the chest, grasp it with the hands and pull it to the chest, then hold for a count of ten. Alternate right and left legs. Repeat four times with each leg.

Round Shoulders, Sunken Chest, Kyphosis, and Protruding Scapulae

Corner Exercise (stretches pectorals). Stand in a corner, with the arms bent at the elbows (shoulder level) and parallel with the floor. With the hands against opposite walls, lean into the corner. Repeat five times.

Arm Circles (strengthens upper back and shoulders and stretches pectorals; also for forward head). With the arms raised sideward to level, circle backward four times; then bend the arms at the elbows and push backward, bringing the shoulder blades together for a count of eight backward movements. Keep the chin tucked and the neck extended; do not allow the head to thrust forward.

Prone Arm Raise (strengthens upper back and shoulders). Lie in a prone position on the floor, with the arms stretched out in front. Raise arms straight toward the ceiling—first left, then right, then both. Repeat the three movements five times.

Back Stroke (strengthens upper back and shoulders). Place the back of the right hand on the right side of the face; press the elbow straight back. Keeping the elbow back, reach backwards with the right hand. Alternate left and right four times on each side, as in swimming the back crawl.

Forward Head

Wall Press (strengthens neck muscles). Stand with your back to the wall with the heels two or three inches from the wall. Press the back of your head against the wall, keep the chin down, and do not increase the lumbar curve. Hold for a count of four, relax for five counts, and repeat three or four times.

Finger Press (strengthens neck muscles). Interlace the fingers behind the head. Pull down with the arms as you push back with the head. Hold for a count of five, relax for five counts, and repeat three or four times.

Head Lift (strengthens neck muscles). Lie in a prone position, with hands clasped behind the head. Apply slight resistance with hands while raising head from the floor. Hold for a count of five, then relax. Repeat five times.

Scoliosis*

(S curve with left dorsal and right lumbar curves. If curves are opposite, reverse the exercise position.)

Bar Hang (stretching). Hang from rings or a bar by the hands with the arms fully extended.

Prone Stretch. Lie prone. Stretch the right arm over head and at the same time stretch the left arm downward and across the back. Hold this position for 30 seconds.

Supine stretch. Lie supine. Draw both knees to the chest and clasp the hands around the knees. Hold this position for 30 seconds.

Scoliosis*

(C curve to the left. If the curve is to the right, reverse the exercises.)

Bar Hang. (see Scoliosis, S curve.)

Stretch Down. Stand with the hands on the hips. Stretch the left arm down at the side and push down firmly. Do not bend the body toward the left side. Repeat five or six times.

Overhead Stretch. Stand with the hands on the hips. Stretch the right arm up overhead; press the left hand against the rib cage at a point which forces the spine into a straighter position. Repeat five or six times.

Flat Back

Shoulder Lift (strengthens muscles in lower back). Lie prone. Place the hands behind the neck, raise the shoulders off the floor, arch the back, keep the hips in contact with the floor.

---

*If you have scoliosis see your physician and perform these exercises only with physician approval.

Lumbar Arch (strengthens muscles in lower back). Stand. Interlock the fingers behind the back in the lumbar area. Press the elbows down and back; try to bring the elbows together. Arch the back in the lumbar area.

Care of the Back and Body Mechanics in Daily Living

7

The spine must support much of the body weight as well as absorb shock and provide for a wide range of trunk movements. These functions are made possible by a flexible backbone composed of twenty-four separate vertebrae plus the sacrum and coccyx, with discs of cartilage between them to absorb shock and prevent friction. While such an arrangement does allow for weight bearing and movement, this same archi-

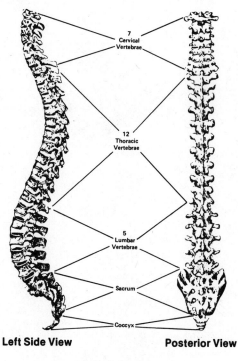

7
Cervical
Vertebrae

12
Thoracic
Vertebrae

5
Lumbar
Vertebrae

Sacrum

Coccyx

Left Side View   **Posterior View**

Spinal Column

tecture makes the back susceptible to strain and injury. "Oh, my aching back!" is a common complaint that afflicts an estimated 75 million Americans and causes a loss of 93 million workdays a year. Its victims spend 35 billion dollars a year for treatments and tests.

According to many authorities, at the rate back pain is increasing, more people will suffer from chronic and recurrent back problems than from any other single medical ailment. Ninety-five percent of all backaches occur in the lower spine. This area sustains the greatest stress from bending and improper posture during sitting and standing.

Causes of Backaches

There are many causes of backaches. Some are actually unrelated to the back, such as kidney disease, peptic ulcer, tipped uterus, infection of the ovaries, or gall bladder. Some back problems may be caused by hereditary structures. Backaches are sometimes psychosomatic—for example, backaches can be a reaction to stress. Stressful situations may stimulate the adrenal glands, creating a change in the body chemistry causing muscle spasms.

Other causes include arthritis, fatigue produced by malnutrition, muscular weakness resulting from inactivity, muscle strain from sudden or forceful bending or twisting, unequal leg lengths, and osteoporosis. Osteoporosis is a condition in which the spine becomes porous and brittle due to the loss of calcium. This occurs mainly in women during the postmenopausal period because of a hormone imbalance, but it may also occur in men. It is not unusual to see disc problems in the early teens, because rapid growth in childhood may cause the spine to outgrow its muscular support.

The most frequent causes of backaches are fatigue and strain due to improper use of the back in daily activities such as lifting too heavy an object or incorrect lifting. Poor posture often is a contributing factor—especially swayback and head-forward deviations, a swayed back (lordosis) is particularly vulnerable to strain and subject to herniated disc due to the excessive curvature of the lumbar portion of the spine. The head-forward position places strain on the posterior neck muscles and can lead to such symptoms as headaches, cricks, dizziness, and pain reflected in the face, scalp, arms, and chest. Neck strain can contribute to pain in the thoracic and lumbar spine.

As Americans become more sedentary in an increasingly automated society, their backs become more vulnerable to injury. The risks are greater for sedentary persons than for the active laborers; for example, the woman who stops exercising when she becomes pregnant will be more prone to backache because her abdominal muscles will become weak.

Many people have hypersensitive spots in their upper back and shoulder muscles which can become very painful and may cause pain to be referred to other areas of the body. Tension headache may result from this referred pain. The hypersensitive spots are called *Trigger Points*. Tense persons and those who assume static postures for long periods of time (such as typists or students) are very prone to these. Some stretching exercises are included in this chapter to help prevent or relieve these "knots" in your muscles.

Prevention and Treatment

To prevent back problems, avoid strain from poor posture and improper use of the back, and on the positive side, perform strengthening and stretching exercises such as those described in this chapter. The chief support for the lower back is the *abdominal muscles*. These must be strengthened along with all other muscles which aid in good posture; these include the *gluteals*—the buttock muscles. The abdominals pull the pelvis up in front and the gluteals pull the pelvis down in back, reducing pelvic tilt. The *back extensor muscles* provide posterior support, while the *lateral trunk muscles* provide lateral support and motion.

It is important that you understand that these four muscle groups work together and are essential to the proper function of the back. Your preventive exercises should be designed to strengthen these muscles and should be done regularly to maintain them. (See Chapter 3 for additional abdominal and gluteal exercises.)

Those who have lordosis should stretch the muscles in the lumbar region and stretch the hip flexors. For those with low back problems, toe touches should be done in a sitting rather than a standing position, so as to reduce the momentum of the upper body.

When the problem appears to be moderate muscle strain of the lower back, rest, heat, and aspirin usually bring relief. If the pain has not subsided in 2 or 3 days, seek the advice of a physician, preferably an orthopedic specialist. The only cure for a "conventional" bad back, once the original cause is diagnosed and corrected, is physical reconditioning. Exercise can be the tool for rebuilding the back structure. This will mean daily exercise; 15 minutes twice daily is preferred. Start slowly and avoid overdoing at the beginning.

Muscle relaxants can be prescribed for temporary relief, but they do not remove the cause. Lying on a hard floor sometimes helps to relieve the pain. There are also times when complete bed rest is necessary. Exercise or activities may be prescribed by physicians. Swimming may be a good exercise, since the buoyancy of the body in the water removes stress on the back. The crawl and the side strokes are the best; avoid the butterfly because of the jerking motion of the spine.

Prevention of Back Problems

1. Avoid the swayback position at all times by taking such precautions as the following:
   a. To relieve back strain during prolonged standing, prop one foot on a stool, bar, or rail, and alternate the foot which takes the major load. Circulate; do not stand in one place for extended periods of time.
   b. When sitting, keep one or both knees higher than the hips by crossing the legs or using a foot rest, keeping the knees bent.
   c. When lying, keep the knees and hips bent; avoid lying on the abdomen; and when lying on the back, place a pillow or lift under the knees.
   d. When lifting and carrying objects, attempting to move a load which is too heavy, or lifting with a jerk, could cause a hernia (rupture).
   e. When driving, the lumbar curve should be flattened against the car seat. Keeping the knees at or above the hip level will achieve this, relieving stress on the back. Get out of the car every hour or two and walk around for a few minutes. If the tilt of the seat can be altered, change the angle periodically.
2. Prevent neck strain by avoiding the head-forward position. The forward thrust is apt to occur in such activities as card playing, sewing, and studying. Sleeping on a high pillow or reclining while watching TV will also result in neck strain.
3. Try to resist wearing high-heeled shoes or boots. They tilt the pelvis, throwing the spine out of line. If you must wear them, do so for only short periods of time.
4. Be aware of how you carry your wallet or purse. Sitting on a thick wallet in the hip pocket can press on the sciatic nerve. Carrying a heavy purse habitually on the same side of the body can result in neck, shoulder and back pain.
5. Do general exercises involving the entire body to help prevent weak muscles.
6. Get adequate rest, and avoid pushing yourself mentally or physically to the point of overfatigue.

In addition to the above suggestions, you can help avoid backache by such common-sense practices, as "warming up" before engaging in strenuous activity, sleeping on a firm mattress, stretching occasionally to relieve tension while studying at a desk, avoiding sudden, jerky movements of the back, keeping weight down to normal, and observing the rules for good body mechanics described throughout this book.

Body Mechanics in Daily Living

Lifting, carrying, pushing, and pulling are normal, everyday activities. It is important to perform them in a correct manner in order to be more efficient, while protecting joints and muscles from undue strain. The avoidance of strain, especially of the back, is the prime consideration in these activities. Some suggestions are given below to aid you in attaining this objective.

Lifting and Carrying

Improper methods of lifting and carrying may cause strain, especially to the lower back. The best method of lifting and carrying a given object will depend upon its weight, mass, and shape. However, the following principles for *lifting* are applicable at all times:

1. Stand close to the object, either in a forward-stride position, with the object at the side, or a side-stride position, with the object between the knees. In the side-stride position, the object is closer to the center of gravity and the lift is straight upward. (See illustration).
2. Keep your back erect, and bend at the hips and knees.
3. Lower your body only as far as necessary, directly downward.
4. Grasp the object and lift with your leg muscles by extending the legs, keeping the object close to your body. Do not lift with a "jerk."
5. Reverse the procedure when lowering the object.
6. Push or pull heavy objects, if this can be done efficiently, rather than lifting them. A good guideline for women is to lift no more than one-third of their body weight. Men should generally lift no more than one-half their body weight. (See illustration next page.)

Some suggestions for *carrying* objects are:

1. Keep the object close to the body's center of gravity.
2. Divide the load, if possible, carrying half in each arm.
3. If the load cannot be divided, occasionally alternate the load from one side of the body to the other.
4. Extend the opposite arm for balance, or lean away from the load.

5. When carrying books—a common activity for students—some faults to be avoided are:
   a. Always carrying books on the same side. This tends to cause the shoulder to be higher than the other and may lead to scoliosis.
   b. Carrying the books in front of the chest. You may have a tendency to lean back to compensate for the additional weight or to hunch forward as you wrap your arms around the books. These actions make the posture unattractive and place a strain on the back.

   Preferably, books should be carried in a brief case or back pack and should be divided equally between both arms. The principles for carrying books also apply when carrying the baby, laundry, grocery sacks, and other loads.
6. Some cautions for *lifting* and *carrying* are:
   a. Do not try to lift or carry loads too heavy for you.
   b. To minimize lower back strain, do not lift or carry heavy objects higher than waist level, except when carrying on the shoulder or head.

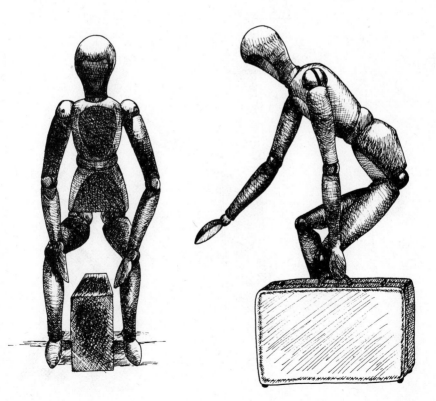

Pulling and Pushing

The best method for *pushing* or *pulling* a given object will depend upon its weight, mass, resistance, and shape, but some general tips are:

1. Keep the back as straight as possible.
2. Use a wide base for balance (stride position).
3. Grasp the object firmly, with the arms fully extended.
4. Bend at the hips and knees, letting the leg muscles do the work.
5. Alternate muscles used by changing the direction you face, such as backward, forward, or sideward.
6. Lean forward from the ankles so that the center of gravity is ahead of the pushing foot.
7. Put glass or metal coasters under heavy furniture to ease the task where friction is great.
8. "Walk" objects too heavy to be moved, such as a refrigerator or couch, by applying force alternately, at one end then the other, in a rotating ("walking") motion.

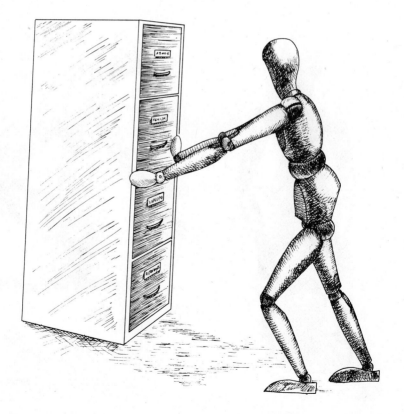

9. Pull a low object with a long handle or rope to make the task easier.

Practicing proper body mechanics in the daily tasks mentioned in the preceding paragraphs will not only help you to avoid strain but will help you to conserve energy for other activities.

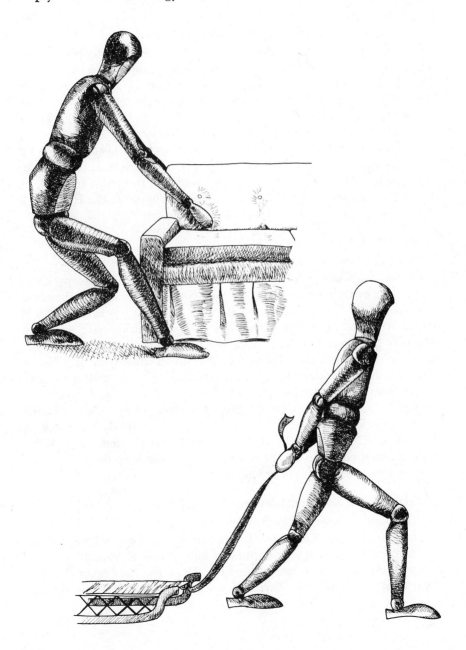

Selected Back Exercises

(Also see abdominal exercises, Chapter 3 and relaxation exercises, Chapter 9).

To Strengthen Upper Back

(Also see exercises for kyphosis, Chapter 3).

Prone Back Lift. Lie prone (face down), with hands clasped behind your neck. Pull your shoulder blades together, raising the elbows off the floor. Slowly raise your head and chest off the floor by arching the upper back. Hold this position for 3 seconds, then slowly return to the starting position. Repeat 10 times. Caution: do not arch the lower back; lift only until the sternum (breastbone) clears the floor.

Isometric Push Back. Tailor sit or stand, with the head up, chin in, elbows raised to shoulder level, fingertips placed on the back of the neck. Push the head and neck backward; and push the fingertips forward, as the elbows are forced backward to flatten the upper back. Hold for 5 or 6 seconds, and then relax. Repeat 2 or 3 times per day.

To Strengthen Lower Back

(not desirable for those with lordosis)

Prone Back and Leg Lift. Same as the prone back lift except, keeping the legs extended, raise them off the floor at the same time the chest is raised. Let the upper and lower back arch. Note: As a general rule, it is best to avoid arching (hyperextending) the lower back during exercises, especially for those with lordosis or low back pain. The prone back lift and the prone back and leg lift may be performed while lying on a bench with the trunk and/or legs hanging over the end. Lift only until the trunk/legs are parallel with the floor).

Limb Lift. Lie in a prone position, with the arms extended overhead and with the legs straight. Slowly lift an arm and leg on the same side of the body as high as possible. Hold for 3 or 4 seconds, and lower slowly to the starting position. Do not roll the body away from the side that is lifted. Alternating sides, repeat 8 times.

To Stretch Lower Back and Alleviate Low Back Pain

(Also see exercises for lordosis, page 60)

Lumbar Stretch. Lie supine (on the back), with knees bent and the feet flat on the floor near your buttocks. Contract your abdominal muscles, flattening the lower back against the floor. Draw one knee up, and pull it down tightly against your chest with your arms. Return to the starting position, then repeat with the other leg. Repeat with each leg 10 to 20 times. When this exercise becomes easy, progress to raising both knees at the same time. For an even greater stretch, try to pull the knees to the axillae (armpits). Combine lumbar stretching with abdominal-strengthening exercises to alleviate low back pain and lordosis.

Rock-A-Bye. Lie supine, draw both knees to the chest, and wrap your arms around the lower legs to bring them close to the trunk. Rock forward and backward as though you were trying to come to a sitting position. Rock four or five times, relax, and repeat three times.

Sit and Reach. Sit with the knees extended and the feet together. Reach forward and grasp your ankles, pulling the trunk forward; hold five seconds. Relax, and repeat three times.

Sit and Curl. Sit in chair and bend forward and hug knees.

To Stretch Trigger Points in Upper Back and Neck

Neck Rotation. Point left fingers toward left ear and place palm of hand against jaw; push head toward right while resisting by trying to rotate head to left; hold isometrically for 4 seconds, then turn head right as far as possible and hold for 4 seconds. Perform exercise 4 times then repeat in other direction 4 times. Do this exercise 4 times daily.

Arm Stretch. Face wall and extend both arms forward to shoulder level, with fingers 6 to 8 inches from wall. Swing the right arm down and around in a big circle, then reach as far forward as possible, trying to touch the wall with the right fingers, without turning your trunk. Hold 4 seconds. Repeat 4 times on each side, 4 times daily.

Rib Separator. Stand with weight on left foot and drop right hip; grasp hands above and behind the head. Bend upper trunk to left and use left arm to pull right arm to left as far as possible. Hold for 4 seconds. Repeat 4 times on each side, 4 times daily. You should feel a stretch under your arm and down the side of your ribs.

Care of the Feet

8

Are you included in the 80 percent of the adult population who complain of foot problems? This is a startling figure, especially since almost 99 percent all feet are perfect at birth. Most of the problems can be prevented or cured by following some basic rules of foot health.

The foot is a complicated structure. Each foot contains 26 bones, 197 ligaments, 19 muscles (18 in the sole alone), and 33 joints. The 14 toe bones are called phalanges; the 5 bones that make up the midfoot are called metatarsals, and the 7 irregular bones in the back of the foot are called tarsals. The main purposes of the feet are weight bearing and locomotion. The number of arches in the foot has been debated by different authorities. Some say there are 3; some 4, while others contend only 2. The most familiar is the longitudinal arch, which runs from the base of the first phalanx to the heel. The function of this arch is to carry weight and absorb the shock of walking. Some writers consider this arch as 2

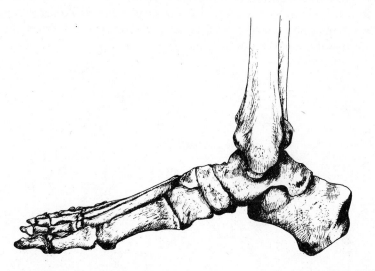

separate arches—the inner and outer longitudinals. The metatarsal arch runs laterally across the ball of the foot and helps to give balance when walking on uneven terrain.

Selection of Footwear

The majority of foot problems are caused by improper shoes or improper use of the foot. If the cause is improperly fitting shoes, the first step in combating the problem is to discard the shoes.

Shoes should never be handed down from person to person if a correct fit is desired. The two most common mistakes made in buying shoes are getting them too narrow or too short. Shoes should be at least half an inch longer than the longest toe. There should be room for the toes to spread out. The ball of the foot should fall over the widest part of the shoe. Try to buy shoes in the late afternoon, when the foot may be as much as a full size larger than it was early in the day. New shoes should be "broken-in" by wearing them for short periods before extended wear such as all day shopping trips. Avoid platform shoes or high heeled (over two inches) shoes or boots, inflexible soles, and pointed-toed shoes. High heels change the center of gravity which puts strain on the metatarsal arch. Leather shoes which lace are almost unbeatable for support. They hug the foot, give with the foot, absorb shock, and allow the foot to breathe.

Shoes for Jogging

Shoes are the only major equipment investment essential for the jogger. They have a more direct effect on the pleasure, performance, and health of the runner than any other factor, including training, since a runner cannot train freely on painful feet. You need to know the difference between good shoes and merely pretty ones.

According to Dr. Harry Hlavac, chief podiatrist at the Sports Clinic in San Francisco, shoes are for protection, support, traction, cushioning from the ground, balance of foot deformities, and the accommodation of foot injuries. Dr. Hlavac says people with normal feet and no injuries are able to wear almost any type of shoes with no pain or disability; but if a person has recurrent problems, then certain types of shoes may help and other types of shoes may aggravate them. For instance, a runner who is susceptible to Achilles tendonitis requires a flexible shoe with cushioning of the bottom of the heel and good elevation. A person with weak ankles and instability needs a shoe that will provide support and balance at heel contact. Calluses on the bottom of the foot require good cushioning. Corns on the top of the foot require a deep toe box and proper fit.

When buying shoes, if one foot is larger than the other, choose the larger size. Use the "standing" rather than the "sitting" size of the foot. Try the shoes on with sports socks and bounce around in them to see how they fit. If the shoe is a correct fit it should need no breaking in. A jogging shoe should not be used for other sports activities because the elevated heel makes the foot slide forward in the shoe when doing quick stops (such as used in basketball and tennis). Also, rippled soles are better for jogging and running, while the nubbed, plain, and herringbone soles are better suited for other activities.

The Runners World magazine asked physicians at the Sports Clinic at the California College of Podiatric Medicine to rate more than 100 different shoe models, looking for the perfect shoe. Their conclusions are listed here.

Good jogging shoes should have these features:*

Sole Makeup—A tough outer layer of rubber with a softer layer under it, totaling a thickness of at least a half-inch.

Sole Bend—The sole can be bent at the forefoot with finger pressure at the end of the shoe.

Heel Width—"Flared" heels (wide, stable platform) have the advantage of extra cushioning. A good shoe measures more than three inches wide at the heel.

Shank Support—The shank is the area under the arch. The shank should be rigid and lie flush with the ground (wedge sole instead of an open area).

Heel Lift—The elevated heel relieves strain on the calf muscles. The heel should have one-half inch more thickness than the sole. It is even better if the heels are rounded up the back.

Inside Support—The shoe should have built-in arch supports, and heel counters (cup around the heel), or both. The need for arch supports is debatable, but manufacturers assume they work.

Upper Softness—Nylon uppers are the best. Leather, including suede has a tendency to grow brittle from weathering and age. A brittle shoe can cause blistering.

Weight—Each shoe should weigh less than 11 ounces.

Width—If you have extremely narrow or wide feet this is important. Different widths are available in some brands.

Features such as breathability, traction, and stability are also considered important. *The Runners World* publishes a "Shoe Issue" each October.

*Reprinted with permission of *Runner's World* in the "Shoe Issue" (October, 1976, p. 38) and October, 1980.

Common Foot Problems

It may be easier, and much wiser, to prevent foot problems than to treat them. Feet should be washed daily and dried carefully. Socks help prevent friction, absorb shock and perspiration. They should be one-fourth inch longer than the longest toe. Cotton or wool materials are very absorbent and are good for feet that perspire heavily.

When walking, one should contact the ground first with the heel, then the outer border of the foot, then the ball of the foot, and finally push off with the toes. Toes should be straight ahead. Toeing out (slue foot) may lead to pronation.

In addition to proper footwear, proper use of the feet, and foot exercises, it may be necessary for some people to have corrective devices (orthotics) prescribed by the physician or podiatrist to alleviate certain foot problems.

Some common foot problems are:

Hard and Soft Corns—Corns are caused by improperly fitting shoes and hose. They can often be relieved by corn pads, or in the case of a soft corn, the use of lamb's wool between the toes. If the corns persist, see your physician or podiatrist (a person who specializes in treating diseases, injuries, and defects of the feet). Do not be a bathroom surgeon; never use corn salves or drops because the caustic acid may injure the surrounding skin.

Calluses—Calluses are caused by friction due to improperly fitting shoes. We sometimes find "loafer's knots" on the heel resulting from loosely fitting shoes rubbing the heel.

Bunions—A chronic inflammation of the bursa sac, bunions are usually found on the joint of the first phalanx. This is caused by pressure and rubbing of the shoe and is aggravated by short, pointed shoes, short or stretch hose, and high heels. Bunions can be relieved by wearing wider shoes, preferably of soft leather. Surgical correction is sometimes necessary because the toe becomes partially dislocated (Hallux Valgus).

. . . **Ingrown Toenails**—Ingrown toenails are the result of cutting the toenails curved instead of straight across, and of improperly fitting shoes and hose. The nail cuts into the skin causing pain and the possibility of infection. This condition usually requires professional care.

Athlete's Foot—Athlete's foot is a fungus infection which usually appears between the toes. It thrives under warm, moist conditions, so the best prevention is to keep the feet clean, dry, and powdered. It may be necessary to change your shoes and hose more than once daily. Rubber thongs can help protect your feet in public bathing or swimming areas.

Crooked or Overlapping Toes—Deformed toes may result from shoes too short or narrow and hose that are too short or of the stretch type. Sometimes, toe deformities are congenital in origin.

Bromidrosis—Bromidrosis is excessive perspiration and odor. Use the same treatment as for athlete's foot. Avoid prolonged wearing of canvas shoes. Antiperspirant deodorant sprays may be helpful.

Plantar Warts—These painful growths that appear on the soles of the feet are caused by a virus and may be transmitted from place to place and person to person. They should be treated by a physician or podiatrist.

Poor Circulation and Fatigue—Poor circulation and fatigue result from long standing and strenous use. Some relief may be obtained by elevating the feet, massage, and contrast baths.

Shortened Achilles Tendon—A shortened Achilles tendon ("heel cord") is caused by constant wearing of high heels, which makes it uncomfortable to wear "flats." The means of correction is to stretch the tendon through exercise (see exercises on page 113.)

Weak Foot Condition

Some symptoms of weak feet are pain in the arch, calf, and lower back; pronation; and general fatigue. Pronation occurs when the weight is borne on the inner border of the foot. The longitudinal arch is lowered and the inner ankle bone protrudes. The Achilles tendon fails to retain the normal vertical line.

Some doctors believe faulty anatomical structure, such as a too-short first metatarsal, can be blamed for some foot weaknesses. Other causes

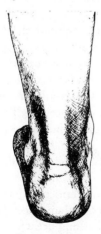

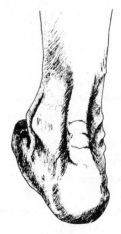

Strong Position   **Pronation**

of weak feet are overweight, muscle strain, disease, congenital defects, inactivity or excessive use, and injury. Use Chart X in the Appendix for a foot evaluation.

Shin Splints

Shin splints are a dull throbbing pain on the shin bone. No one really knows what causes them. Some theories are that shin splints are caused by changing running surfaces (hard to soft), running on hard surfaces, bringing one foot over too much in front of the other one when running (putting pressure on the fibula), wearing improper shoes, being overweight, or using the feet and legs in an unaccustomed manner such as overuse or improper use. Some pathological theories are that the muscle has pulled away from the bone, the membrane between the tibia and fibula is stretched, or that there are microscopic tears in the muscles.

Shin splints are more likely to occur in a person whose muscles are weak. The only cure is rest. Several different treatments might alleviate the pain, such as the application of cold or heat, massage, or a combination of these. Shin splints are a very individual condition; thus what works for one person may not help another. Stretching the calf muscles and strengthening the anterior tibial muscles may help prevent shin splints. Stretching the shin muscles before and after, jogging may also help prevent or alleviate the pain. Many people tape the tibia and fibula together but, this is not a good practice since it can retard circulation to the foot.

Selected Foot Exercises

1. **Toe Curling**—Curling the toes improves circulation (a big factor in preventing varicose veins) and strengthens the arches.
2. **Walking Barefoot in the Sand**—This is a good exercise for foot muscles.
3. **Outward Roll**—Stand with the feet slightly apart and roll the weight toward the outside borders of the feet. Repeat 10 times.
4. **Walk on Tiptoes**—Walk with the feet toeing in (pigeon toed) for 50 steps.
5. **Marble Pickup**—Pick up marbles or an imaginary object with your toes. Repeat 10 times.
6. **Achilles Stretch**—Stand with the toes and balls of the feet on a thick book. Lower the heels to the floor. Repeat 10 times.
7. **Foot Circling**—Sit, or lie supine, with the legs extended. Point the toes of the feet downward, turn the soles toward each other, bring the toes toward the shins (dorsiflex). Repeat 10 times.

8. **Towel Grip**—Sit on a stool or chair and place a towel on the floor. Keep the feet parallel (about 10 inches apart) and under the knees. Grip the towel with the toes and gather it into a mound.
9. **Isometric Inversion**—Sit in a chair with one ankle resting on the other thigh. Supinate the foot while resisting with the hands.
10. **Shin Stretch**—Sit in chair and extend both legs in front of body, keeping feet flat on floor, force the ankles into plantar flexion, stretching the anterior tibialis.

Relaxation

9

Relaxation may be defined as the release of neuromuscular tension. It is a skill which can be learned and practiced and is as important an aspect of total fitness as is strength. Unfortunately, it is an aspect too often neglected. With the present-day emphasis on contracting muscles, we forget to learn how to "uncontract" them.

We are faced daily with tension-building situations in this fast-paced modern world. The game of the century is "Beat the Clock"—competition under pressure, and a race against time. We build up tension from worry, fears, anxiety, and physical and mental fatigue. We need ways to prevent or release these tensions; therefore, relaxation plays a vital part in contributing to one's health.

Tension

Tension is necessary in order to be awake and alert. It is a general condition of activity in the body—a state of "readiness" for response on the part of the muscles, organs, glands, and nerves. What we are concerned about is *excess* tension: specifically, residual neuromuscular hypertension. Failure to release unnecessary tensions because of inadequate rest and sleep, and the inability to relax will result in a chronic state of fatigue and excess muscle tension. This muscle tension may cause backaches, headaches, or difficulty in getting to sleep. Heart attacks, ulcers, menstrual irregularities, nervous, and psychic disorders may be related to conditions of tension.

Tension may manifest itself in nervous mannerisms such as fidgeting and finger tapping; or in static positions such as clenched teeth, frowning, and a tight fist. Incoordination and inefficiency, as well as psychosomatic ailments such as headaches and digestive upsets, may be symptomatic of neuromuscular hypertension.

Dr. Roy Menninger, the noted psychiatrist, states that 70 per cent of the population are affected from time to time with "problems of living." He contends that stress need not be bad for people. Many persons actually thrive on stress. The problem is learning to cope with stress. Dr. Menninger says that people must recognize stress and train themselves to withdraw temporarily from the circumstances.

Prevention of Neuromuscular Hypertension

Much tension can be avoided by proper planning of your daily life—balancing work and rest. "Moderation in all things" may still be a helpful adage. At the first sign of fatigue, when you feel yourself becoming irritable, take a "breather." Provision should be made for recreational activities and diversions which promote the release of inner stresses. Whether it be a rousing game of tennis, gardening, or music, one needs a "safety valve" to prevent built-up tension. Good body mechanics can help to prevent tension, since efficient movement requires the use of only those muscles essential to the task, preventing unnecessary energy expenditure and strain.

Methods of Releasing Tension

Alcohol, tranquilizers, pain pills, and other drugs are not the answer. Begin by trying to find out why you are tense, and strive to remove the cause. Some people can relax more easily than others; but releasing tension is a matter of self-discipline and can be learned.

Recreation, in the out-of-doors if possible, is strongly recommended as both a sedative and a cathartic. Massage and heat are soothing and comforting. Mild, rhythmic exercise routines can be beneficial. Stretching exercises to pull the tightness out of muscles are good if done slowly and held for a moment. Try rolling your head in a large circle on your shoulders. As a break from your studies, lie with your feet elevated and your neck supported by a rolled-up towel for 10 or 15 minutes.

It is not uncommon to find it difficult to reduce body tensions enough to fall asleep at night. Some suggestions for preventing this "wide-eyed" feeling are:

1. Go to bed at a regular time.
2. Avoid eating *heavy* foods before bedtime.
3. Start "letting down" at least 45 minutes before retiring.
4. Take a warm shower.
5. Eliminate distractions such as light and noise.

Conscious Techniques of Relaxation

A conscious relaxation of at least 20 minutes a day is remarkably helpful. Use of such a technique before falling asleep will help insure falling asleep more quickly, and result in a sounder, more restful sleep. There are a number of well-known "methods" of relaxing, and while these systems differ somewhat, most of them offer suggestions similar to these:

1. Learn to recognize neuromuscular tension in a body part and the feeling of releasing it by deliberately tightening a muscle and then "leting it go." Relaxing is said to be zero activity—not something you do, but rather, something you cease to do.
2. Lie on your back in a comfortable position, and concentrate on your breathing without changing its rhythm. Gradually extend the exhalation, and as you do so, consciously release the muscular tension in your body.
3. Try to "let go," and continue "letting go" beyond the point of zero tension. Start at the toes (or some other body part) and work up to the legs, thighs, abdomen, lower back, upper back, arms, neck, shoulders, chest, face, mouth, jaw, and tongue. It is easier to relax the large muscle groups (arms, legs, trunk, and neck), but with practice, the small muscles (face, mouth, and tongue) can also be controlled.
4. Success may not be immediate, but it will come with practice. As skill is acquired, you may be able to release tension in the body as a whole rather than concentrating on individual body parts.
5. Use a "sort-of" self-hypnosis, imagining yourself on a feather bed or floating on a cloud; or visualizing yourself as a rag doll or a heavy bag of sand, with the sand slowly sifting through a hole in the sack.

Several popular exercise and relaxation systems follow patterns similar to those listed. Yoga, Zen, Transcendental Meditation, and other Eastern Groups base a large part of their programs on relaxation techniques.

With practice, and the acquisition of the kinesthetic perception for tension and the release of tension, conscious relaxation can be used in almost any situation where tension builds up in your daily life. Lying, sitting, or standing, you can learn to relax isolated body parts or the entire body when the situation demands and without others noticing your technique. Whether it be final examination jitters or stage fright before an audience, the ability to relax will make your adjustment to life more successful.

Selected Relaxation Exercises

Arm Swings

1. Stand with the feet apart; inhale as the arms are slowly raised forward to shoulder height. Exhale, and release all muscular tension in the arms, allowing them to drop to the sides and swing passively until all momentum is spent.
2. Repeat as above, except raise the arms to the side.
3. Repeat as above, except after the arms drop and swing down and backward and rebound forward, raise them to shoulder height again as you inhale. Repeat pendular relaxed swings in rhythm with your breathing.

Leg Swings

Stand on one leg, with the hip on the opposite side elevated so that the leg can swing freely, just brushing the floor with your foot. Execute leg swings the same as arm swings, using a minimum of muscular contraction, with tension only as the forward momentum is spent and the leg is raised to hip level. Keep the lower leg relaxed and the knee bent on the forward lift.

Trunk Swings

Stand with your feet apart and the knees slightly bent. Bend forward at the hips, and let the head, neck, arms, and trunk dangle toward the floor. With a minimum of muscular effort, set the trunk swinging from side to side by shifting the weight from one foot to the other, letting the heels come off the floor alternately. Then, with a slight springing movement of the lower back, gently bob up and down, keeping the entire body limp.

Shoulder Drop

Sit tailor fashion on the floor, or sit in a chair with arms relaxed. Tip your head back, and let it hang relaxed. Inhale and hunch one shoulder, then let it drop as you exhale; repeat with the other shoulder; repeat with both shoulders at the same time; repeat with the head tipped forward or tipped toward the opposite shoulder.

Menstruation and Pregnancy

10

Menstruation, which begins at puberty and ends at menopause, is a series of events occurring in a cycle. Normally a woman will menstruate four to six days at 20 to 30 day intervals, but it varies with the individual— five days at 28 day interval is average. The purpose of the menstrual cycle is to prepare the uterus for nurturing a new life and to eliminate that preparation if the ovum is not fertilized. The walls of the uterus become engorged with blood and nutritive elements to supply the fertilized ovum with a means of growth. This cannot return to the blood stream and so is lost by a direct flow from the uterus.

The entire cycle is a normal process and should not be painful. However, there are normal biochemical changes occurring in the body during menstruation, such as increased congestion in the pelvic area, heightened irritability, lowered threshold for pain, more susceptibility to environmental temperature changes, and decreased flexibility (especially in the lower back and pelvic regions). Common symptoms, preceding and during the menstrual flow, may be one or more of the following: protruding abdomen, enlarged breasts and soreness, weight gain, and pain (cramps, headache, leg ache, nausea and low back pain). Changes in one's daily routine, such as emotional upsets and new living arrangements, can result in minor fluctuations in the cycle.

Dysmenorrhea

Dysmenorrhea (painful menstruation) is not normal, but approximately one-half of the women who menstruate have menstrual discomfort with some regularity. Many have severe pain that incapacitates them for a day or two each month. It is one of the most common causes of lost work and school hours in the country; 140 million work hours are lost each year. Loss of work time because of this so-called "feminine handicap" has been a problem for employers and labor unions.[1]

119

There are two general types—structural and functional. Structural dysmenorrhea arises from such things as malformations, endocrine imbalance, or malpositions and should be referred to your family doctor for diagnosis and treatment. Innumerable theories have been advanced as to the causes of functional dysmenorrhea: defective posture (especially swayback), fatigue, tension, constipation, lack of muscle tone, and sluggish circulation due to lack of exercise. Gynecologists estimate that seventy to eighty percent of the cases of painful menstruation are functional.

Recent research has determined that there are at least ten prescription drugs that are effective in the majority of cases of dysmenorrhea. These are anti-prostaglandin drugs. Indications show that dysmenorrheic women often have high levels of hormone-like proteins called prostaglandins. According to current thinking, raised levels of prostaglandins produced by many tissues of the body (including uterus lining) cause contractions, lack of oxygen, and nervous sensitivity which create dysmenorrhea in some women. Prostaglandin inhibitors are marketed primarily as anti-inflammatory drugs for arthritis. Since these drugs are taken for so short a period, the side effects so far have been minimal. Aspirin, also inhibits prostaglandins, but is much weaker than the prescription drugs. Any woman with severe menstrual cramps should discuss this treatment with her physician.

You may prevent or find relief from minor pain by:

1. Improving your daily health habits through an adequate diet and a balance of activity and rest.
2. Improving poor posture.
3. Exercising regularly and using special remedial exercises.
4. Wearing proper clothing (avoid tight belts and girdles).
5. Applying heat to the lower back and abdomen.
6. Learning to relax (see Chapter 9).

A large majority of gynecologists place no restrictions on the usual daily routine, including vigorous activity (such as swimming) and intensive sports competition during all phases of the cycle. Normal hygiene practices should be carried on—bathing, shampooing hair, etc. It is extremely important that you observe care in your personal cleanliness while menstruating because you may perspire more and body odors are more offensive at this time—even your breath may carry a distinctive menstrual odor.

Selected Exercises for Dysmenorrhea

Many exercises or physical activities that improve circulation and lower back flexibility may prevent dysmenorrhea or give relief. A few of the exercises, some named for the gynecologists by whom they were prescribed, are described below:

Billig Exercise. Stand with your left side to the wall, heels and toes together; left arm bent at a right angle, forearm and hand resting on the wall at shoulder level parallel to the floor. Place the right hand on the right hip; and "push" the hips slowly and steadily toward the wall, keeping the back erect, lower back flat, and the knees extended. Do this 3 times to the left and 3 times to the right. Repeat 3 times a day.

Mosher Exercise. Assume a hook-lying position, with the right hand resting on the abdomen. Raise the lower abdomen as high as possible (balloon), keeping the lower back flat on the floor. Lower the abdomen by pulling in and up and contracting your abdominals. Repeat 10 to 20 times. Do not hold your breath but continue to breathe normally.

Knee-Chest Position. Kneel with the thighs perpendicular to the floor, rest the cheek on the floor, and place your arms at your sides or place your hands under the cheek. Maintain this position for 10 to 15 minutes.

Mad Cat Exercise. On hands and knees with head raised permit the abdominals "to drop" and the back to sway. Then drop the head and flatten the abdomen by "pulling it in," and "hump" the back, holding for a count of 5. Relax for 5 counts and repeat 3 or 4 times.

Exercises for the Pregnant Woman

Normally, you should continue to be physically active during pregnancy. Exercise during this period and after giving birth is as essential to good health as under ordinary circumstances. With regular exercise, you will not only feel better but also be better prepared for the delivery of your baby. Many daily activities such as sitting, standing, walking, stair climbing, kneeling, and squatting are good forms of exercise. Since these activities compose a much greater percentage of your movements during the day than a regular exercise routine, they should be performed with efficient body mechanics. You should consult your doctor before undertaking or continuing an exercise program during pregnancy.

Selected Exercises for the Pregnant Woman

Leg Extensor–Assume a hook-lying position. Slowly slide the right leg down, keeping the sole of the foot and the base of the spine on the floor as long as possible. Extend the leg fully, and then slowly slide the leg to the initial position. Repeat 3 to 5 times with each leg. Inhaling as the foot slides up and exhaling as it slides down.

Knee Raise—Assume a hook-lying position. Bring the right thigh toward the chest, keeping the knee bent. Return to the initial position, and repeat with the other leg. Repeat 3 to 5 times with each leg, inhaling as the thigh comes up and exhaling as it goes down.

Frog Kick—Lie supine. Place soles of feet together by rotating legs outward. Draw the legs upward until the outsides of the knees are touching, or almost touching, the floor. Extend legs downward, keeping the soles of the feet together as long as you can. Repeat slowly 3 to 5 times, inhaling as legs are drawn upward and exhaling as they are extended.

Hip Raiser—Assume a hook-lying position, with arms at sides. Slowly raise the lower part of the spine off the floor as the body weight is shifted toward your knees and heels as if trying to get up. Gradually return to the initial position, leading with the lower part of your spine. Repeat 3 to 5 times, inhaling as the spine is raised and exhaling as it is lowered.

Back Relaxer—Assume a supine position with arms at sides. Sit up; grasp your right knee, keeping the left leg extended. Keep the left leg on the floor as you rock back and forth 5 or 6 times, holding the right knee. Return to the initial position, and repeat with the left knee. Keep your back curved and your breathing effortless.

Leg Relaxer—Lie supine. Place your lower legs on a chair or stool of average height. Heels should be fully supported and the chair placed so that you have no feeling of holding up your legs. Relax. Take deep breaths through your nose and exhale through your mouth.

Ankle Flex—Lie supine with legs extended, arms at sides. Flex your ankles by pointing with the heels. Repeat 10 to 12 times, inhaling as you flex and exhaling on the return to initial position.

Arm Twist—Stand erect, facing a wall at about an arm's length. Place the palms of your hands on the wall directly in front of your shoulders. Lean forward slightly, resting your weight on both hands. Without moving, your hands, rotate the elbows until they point outward, and then return to initial position. Repeat slowly 5 or 6 times. Place your hands so that the fngertips point toward one another. Rotate the elbows downward and then return to initial position. Repeat slowly 5 or 6 times, exhaling as elbows go down and inhaling as they go up.

Other Menstrual Conditions

Toxic Shock Syndrome—Although rare, this syndrome is of concern to some tampon users. This disease is caused by a bacterium, Staphylococcus Aureus. The part tampons play in this is not yet known. Medical consultants suggest that if you use tampons do not use them continually; use menstrual pads at night and on days of light flow.

Secondary Amenorrhea—Cessation of the menstrual flow, has appeared in females who do intense and frequent aerobic work bouts. Many female distance runners, those who run 10 to 15 miles per day experience this condition, as do some dancers and cyclists. The reason for this is not known, but one theory postulates that there is a correlation between secondary amenorrhea and lowered percentage of body fat. Usually when the intensive work bouts cease the menses returns.

References

1. Sue Miller, "Menstrual Cramps 'not in your head' " *Times-Union and Journal,* Jacksonville, Sunday, January 25, 1981, p. F-6.

Appendix

Charts

CHART I

Tests and Measurements
(tear out)

Name _____ Section _____ Date _____

Wrist _____ Ankle _____ Height _____ Ideal Weight _____

Body Measurements
(measure to nearest 1/8″)

	Initial	Goal	Final	Reached Goal	Improved	Stayed Same	Worsened
Weight	_____	_____	_____				
Bust/Chest	_____	_____	_____				
Waist	_____	_____	_____				
Abdomen	_____	_____	_____				
Hips	_____	_____	_____				
Thigh	_____	_____	_____				
Calf	_____	_____	_____				
Upper Arm	_____	_____	_____				
% Fat	_____	_____	_____				

Physical Fitness

	Pretest			Postest	
	Raw Score	Rank	Goal	Raw Score	Rank
Sit and reach	_____	_____	_____	_____	_____
Sit-ups	_____	_____	_____	_____	_____
Pull-ups/Hang	_____	_____	_____	_____	_____
Push-ups	_____	_____	_____	_____	_____
1.5 mi. run	_____	_____	_____	_____	_____

Final Results

Reached goal _____ Improved _____ Stayed Same _____ Worsened _____

CHART II

Weekly Chart for Weight and Measurements
(tear out)

Name _____ Section _____

	Initial	Goal	Weeks 2	4	6	8	10	12	14	16	Total Change	Reached Goal	Improved	Stayed Same	Worsened
Weight															
Bust/Chest															
Waist															
Abdomen															
Hips															
Thigh															
Calf															
Upper arm															
Skinfold															
Biceps															
Triceps															
Iliac															
Subscapular															
total															
% fat															
rank															

CHART III

Calculate Your Work Capacity

Name _____ Section _____ Date _____

Key

RHR	Resting Heart Rate
MHR	Maximum Heart Rate
HRR	Heart Rate Range
HR	Heart Rate at Working Capacity
40%	Sub-minimal Training
60%	Minimal Training
75%	Maximal Training

Base Information

RHR _____ (beats per minute while sitting)

MHR _____ (220 − your age)

Calculations

for 40% Working Capacity

_____ (MHR) − ____ (RHR) = ____ × .40 + ____ (RHR) = ____ (HR)

for 60% Working Capacity

_____ (MHR) − ____ (RHR) = ____ × .60 + ____ (RHR) = ____ (HR)

for 75% Working Capacity

_____ (MHR) − ____ (RHR) = ____ × .75 + ____ (RHR) = ____ (HR)

Name _J ohn Doe_ _____   Section _9 o'clock M W F_

Goal _20_ _____ in 10 weeks.

CHART IV-A

Graph Your Weight Change
(tear out)

If you are trying to gain or lose, graph your change in weight by plotting it with a "dot" each week. Connect the dots with a straight line. Note: each square represents one pound lost or gained. In the sample, the person lost 20 pounds in 10 weeks. This is a sample for John Doe; use Chart IVB on other side.

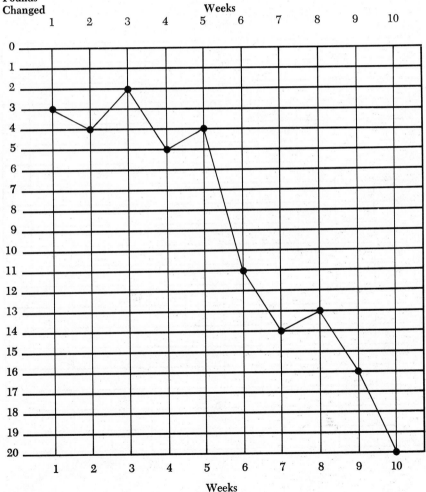

Pounds Changed

Weeks

Weeks

Name ____ Section ________________

Goal ____________ in 10 weeks.

CHART IV-B

Graph Your Weight Change
(tear out)

If you are trying to gain or lose, graph your change in weight by plotting it with a "dot" each week. Connect the dots with a straight line. Note: each square represents one pound lost of gained.

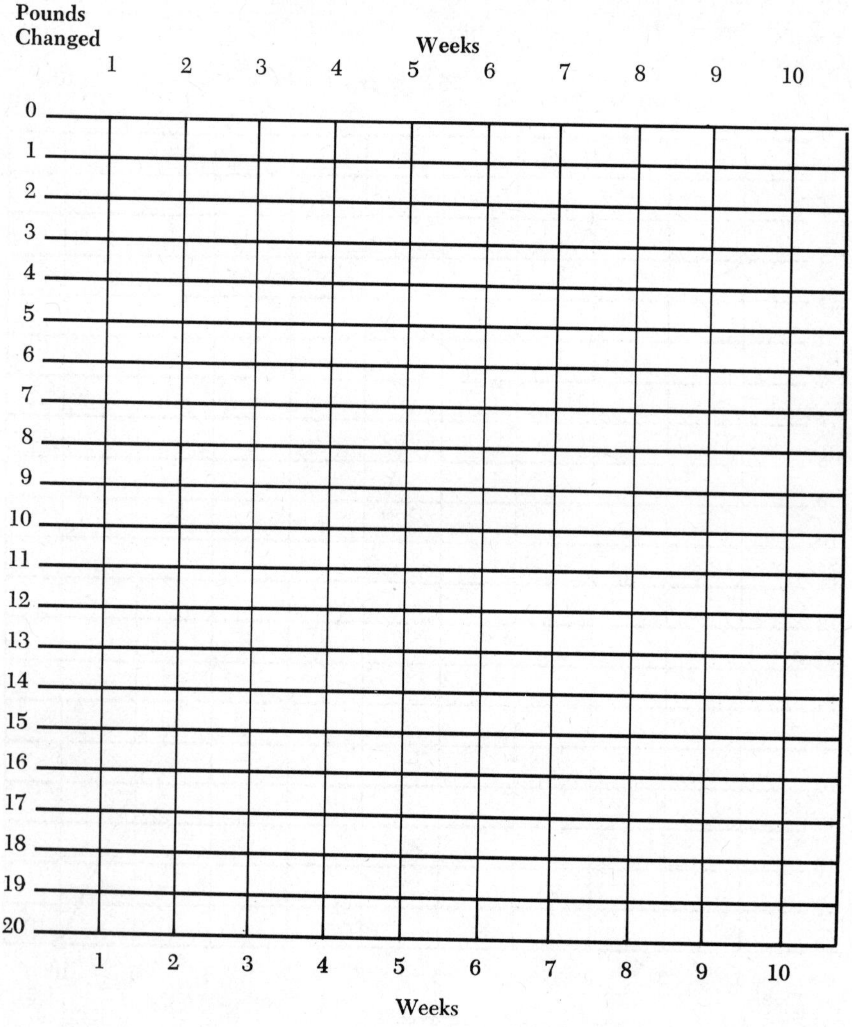
Pounds Changed
Weeks
1 2 3 4 5 6 7 8 9 10
0 1 2 3 4 5 6 7 8 9 10 11 12 13 14 15 16 17 18 19 20
1 2 3 4 5 6 7 8 9 10
Weeks

CHART V-A

What Can I Do About Me?

(tear out)

Name _____ Section _____ Date _____

Having taken inventory of your present status, look at the "shape you're in." Is there room for improvement? Using the chart below, summarize your weaknesses, and set some realistic goals which you will strive to attain. In the left-hand column, diagnose your faults; in the center column, write your prescription (specific exercises, personal habits, etc.) for remedying that weakness; and in the right-hand columns, indicate your goals.

DIAGNOSIS	Yes No	PRESCRIPTION	PROGNOSIS (I can improve)		
			Next Week	Next Mo.	In 6 Mos.
1. Posture Do I have:					
a. A forward head?					
b. Round shoulders?					
c. Sunken chest?					
d. Scoliosis?					
e. Kyphosis?					
f. Lordosis?					
g. Abdominal ptosis?					
h. Hyper-extended knees?					
i. fatigue slump?					
2. Weight Am I:					
a. Overweight?					
b. Underweight?					
c. Malnourished?					

CHART V-B
What Can I Do About Me?
(tear out)

DIAGNOSIS	Yes No	PRESCRIPTION	PROGNOSIS (I can improve)		
			Next Week	Next Mo.	In 6 Mos.
3. Physical Fitness Are my scores above average?					
a. Cardiovascular endurance?					
b. Abdominal strength and endurance?					
c. Arm and shoulder strength and endurance?					
d. Flexibility?					
e. Arm strength and endurance?					
4. Figure/physique: Am I pleased with my:					
a. General appearance?					
b. Bust/Chest?					
c. Waist?					
d. Abdomen?					
e. Hips?					
f. Thigh?					
g. Calf?					
h. Upper arm?					

CHART VI

Test Your Knowledge About Food
and Weight Reduction*
(tear out)

Name_____ **Section** _____ **Date** _____

Circle T for True or F for false.

T   F   1. Hard-boiled eggs are less "fattening" than soft-boiled eggs.

T   F   2. Potato is very fattening.

T   F   3. You will lose fat-weight faster on a high protein diet.

T   F   4. Oleomargarine is less fattening than butter.

T   F   5. You can eat and drink whatever you please if you take a vitamin and
mineral capsule daily.

T   F   6. You can do without sugar and starchy foods equally well, on a weight-
loss diet.

T   F   7. Toasted bread is less fattening than untoasted bread.

T   F   8. Canned vegetables are not as nourishing as fresh vegetables prepared
at home.

T   F   9. Massage is helpful in weight reduction.

T   F   10. Food eaten before you go to bed is more apt to cause weight gain than
the same food eaten for breakfast.

T   F   11. Sweet chocolate is less fattening than bitter.

T   F   12. Milk should be included in a weight-reducing diet.

T   F   13. A good way to cut out calories, is to skip meals while reducing.

T   F   14. Sour cream is less fattening than light sweet cream.

T   F   15. Carbohydrates are more fattening than protein.

T   F   16. Brown sugar is more fattening than white.

T   F   17. Sherbets and ices are less fattening than ice cream.

T   F   18. One should drink less water while on a reducing diet.

T   F   19. Certain foods are "slenderizing."

T   F   20. It makes no difference whether a person eats fast or slow.

*Answers available to the teacher in *The Instructors Handbook*.

CHART VII

Weekly Calorie Summary
(tear out)

Duplicate seven copies of the sample "DAILY CALORIE CHART" (Chart VIII found on the back side of this page). Tear out or duplicate one copy of this page. Record your food intake for one "normal" week. Do not change from your regular eating patterns. Carefully record all foods and amounts and the number of calories. Total for each meal, day and week.

On the chart below, place an X in each box when you have eaten that food group. The number of boxes represents the minimum servings recommended.

	Dairy Products	Meat, Fish and Eggs	Vegetables and Fruits	Breads and Cereals
Monday	☐ ☐	☐ ☐	☐ ☐ ☐ ☐	☐ ☐ ☐ ☐
Tuesday	☐ ☐	☐ ☐	☐ ☐ ☐ ☐	☐ ☐ ☐ ☐
Wednesday	☐ ☐	☐ ☐	☐ ☐ ☐ ☐	☐ ☐ ☐ ☐
Thursday	☐ ☐	☐ ☐	☐ ☐ ☐ ☐	☐ ☐ ☐ ☐
Friday	☐ ☐	☐ ☐	☐ ☐ ☐ ☐	☐ ☐ ☐ ☐
Saturday	☐ ☐	☐ ☐	☐ ☐ ☐ ☐	☐ ☐ ☐ ☐
Sunday	☐ ☐	☐ ☐	☐ ☐ ☐ ☐	☐ ☐ ☐ ☐

lose
Present weight _____ Ideal Weight _____ Pounds to gain _____

Estimated caloric needs to maintain ideal weight (15 × ideal wt.)_____

Actual caloric intake (weeks total ÷ 7)_____

Estimated caloric intake needed to lose/gain one pound per week _____

Did you meet the minimum recommended servings of the four food groups?_____

In what were you deficient?_____

Did you eat one nutrient in excess? What?_____

What changes, if any, should you make in your eating habits on a temporary or permanent basis.

_____

_____

_____

_____

_____

_____

_____

If you decide to gain or lose, you may need to continue counting and recording calories until you reach your goal. Chart IV may be used along with Charts VII & VIII.

CHART VIII

Daily Calorie Chart
(tear out)

Name_____ Section _____ Date _____

Breakfast food	Amount	Calories
		Total Calories _____
Lunch food	Amount	Calories
		Total Calories _____
Dinner food	Amount	Calories
		Total Calories _____
Snack food	Amount	Calories
		Total Calories _____
Daily total intake		

CHART IX

Postural Defects
(tear out)

Number _____

Name_____ Section _____

Number 1 date_____Number 2 Date_____

_____ Head forward _____

_____ Kyphosis _____

_____ Round shoulders _____

_____ Sunken chest _____

_____ Lordosis _____

_____ Flat back _____

_____ Abdominal ptosis _____

_____ Hyper-extended knees _____

_____ Body lean _____

_____ Scoliosis _____

_____ Protruding scapulae _____

_____ Fatigue slump _____

_____ Rating _____

IMPROVEMENT _____

Key: O, no defect   X, slight defect   XX, needs attention   XXX, severe

CHART X

Foot Evaluation
(tear out)

	RIGHT	LEFT
Corns		
Calluses		
Bunions		
Ingrown toenails		
Deformed toes		
Kneecaps in		
Kneecaps out		
Pronation		
Low longitudinal arch		
Low metatarsal arch		
Toeing in		
Toeing out		
Others		

KEY: O, no defect; X, slight; XX, moderate; XXX, severe

Index

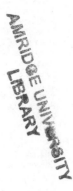